Atlas of Temporomandibular Joint Surgery

Atlas of Temporomandibular Joint Surgery

EDITORS

Peter D. Quinn, DMD, MD

Professor, Department of Oral and Maxillofacial Surgery, University of Pennsylvania School of Dental Medicine
Vice Dean for Professional Services, University of Pennsylvania School of Medicine
Philadelphia, PA, USA

Eric J. Granquist, DMD, MD

Clinical Associate, Department of Oral and Maxillofacial Surgery
Philadelphia, PA, USA

SECOND EDITION

WITH CONTRIBUTION FROM

MEDICAL ILLUSTRATOR PAUL SCHIFFMACHER

WILEY Blackwell

Library of Congress Cataloging-in-Publication Data

Color atlas of temporomandibular joint surgery.
  Atlas of temporomandibular joint surgery / editors, Peter D. Quinn, Eric J. Granquist. – Second edition.
    p. ; cm.
  Preceded by Color atlas of temporomandibular joint surgery / Peter D. Quinn. c1998.
  Includes bibliographical references and index.
  ISBN 978-1-119-94985-5 (cloth)
I. Quinn, Peter D., 1948– , editor. II. Granquist, Eric J., editor. III. Title.
[DNLM: 1. Temporomandibular Joint–surgery–Atlases. 2. Temporomandibular Joint Disorders–surgery–Atlases. WU 17]
  RK529
  617.5′22059–dc23
                                    2014047520

A catalogue record for this book is available from the British Library.

Set in 10/13pt Meridien by SPi Publisher Services, Pondicherry, India

1 2015

Contents

Contributors list, vii

Preface, ix

Acknowledgments, xi

About the companion website, xiii

1 Surgical decision making for temporomandibular joint surgery, 1

2 Diagnostic imaging of the temporomandibular joint, 5

3 Surgical approaches to the temporomandibular joint, 31

4 Surgery for internal derangements, 57

5 Osseous surgery of the temporomandibular joint, 85

6 Trauma, 105

7 Autogenous reconstruction of the temporomandibular joint, 131

8 Stock alloplastic reconstruction of the temporomandibular joint, 145

9 Custom alloplastic reconstruction of the temporomandibular joint, 181

10 Pathology of the temporomandibular joint, 203

11 Complications, 231

Index, 245

Contributors list

Helen Giannakopoulos DDS, MD
Associate Professor, Department
of Oral and Maxillofacial Surgery,
University of Pennsylvania
School of Dental Medicine
Philadelphia, PA, USA

Guo Bai DDS, MD
Resident, Department of Oral Surgery,
Ninth People's Hospital, Shanghai Jiao
Tong University School of Medicine
Shanghai, China

Michael Bowler BDS (Otago, NZ), FDSRCS (Edin.), FFDRCS (Irel.), FICD
Private Practice
Charlestown, NSW, Australia

Ron Caloss DDS, MD
Associate Professor and Chairman,
Department of Oral-Maxillofacial
Surgery, University of Mississippi
Medical Center
Jackson, MS

Lee Carrasco DDS, MD
Associate Professor, Department of Oral
and Maxillofacial Surgery, University of
Pennsylvania School of Dental
Medicine
Philadelphia, PA, USA

David C. Stanton DMD, MD, FACS
Associate Professor, Department
of Oral and Maxillofacial Surgery,
University of Pennsylvania
School of Dental Medicine
Philadelphia, PA, USA

Sotirios Diamantis DMD, MD
Private practice
Lowell, MA, USA

Jan Faulk DDS
Associate Professor, Department of Oral
and Maxillofacial Surgery
University of North Carolina at Chapel
Hill School of Dentistry
Chapel Hill, NC, USA

Paul Henrique Luiz de Freital PhD
Professor, Dental School, Federal
University of Sergipe at Lgarto
Lagarto, Brazil

Dongmei He DDs, MD
Professor, Department of Oral Surgery,
Ninth People's Hospital, Shanghai Jiao
Tong University School of Medicine
Shanghai, China

N. Shaun Matthews BDS, FDS, MBBS, FRCS (Edin), FRCS (OMFS)
Consultant Oral and Maxillofacial Surgeon
King's College Hospital
London, England, UK

Louis G. Mercuri DDS, MS
Visiting Professor, Department of
Orthopedic Surgery
Rush University Medical Center
Chicago, IL, USA

Clinical Consultant
TMJ Concepts
Ventura, CA, USA

Gerhard Undt
Professor
Hospital for Cranio-Maxillofacial and
Oral Surgery
Vienna, Austria

Gary Warburton DDS, MD, FACS
Associate Professor, Department of Oral
and Maxillofacial Surgery, University of
Maryland School of Dentistry
Baltimore, MD, USA

Anders Westermark DDS, PhD
Associate Professor
Aland Central Hospital
Aland, Finland

Larry M. Wolford DMD
Clinical Professor, Department of Oral
and Maxillofacial Surgery and
Orthodontics, Texas A&M University
Health Science Center, Baylor College of
Dentistry, Baylor University Medical
Center
Dallas, TX, USA

Chi Yang DDS, MD
Professor, Department of Oral Surgery,
Ninth People's Hospital, Shanghai Jiao
Tong University School of Medicine
Shanghai, China

Preface

Surgical knowledge depends on long practice, not from speculation.

Marcello Malpighi, 1689

Surgical management of the temporomandibular joint has been one of the most vexing and controversial disciplines within oral and maxillofacial surgery. In 1999, we felt that there had been substantial evidence-based initiatives in therapeutic surgical interventions for advanced temporomandibular joint disorders sufficient enough to warrant a surgical atlas. We believe that the incredible advances over the last 15 years in surgical management, and decision-making, clearly justify an updated edition of this atlas. Both editions presume that a comprehensive, nonsurgical intervention has been explored prior to consideration of any open surgical approach. We wanted to produce a concise "how-to" surgical guide for both the novice and experienced surgeon. Intra-articular and extra-articular open procedures, for the correction of diseases involving the temporomandibular joint, which have been shown to be safe and efficacious are reviewed in detail. We believe that only through clinical trials, and well-designed translational research, will we continue to further our understanding of the complexities of this unique articulation. It is our sincere hope that the second edition of this surgical atlas will contribute to this most important scientific endeavor.

Acknowledgments

To Dr. Louis Schoenleber for his wisdom, mentorship, and generosity.

To our colleagues in the American Society of Temporomandibular Surgeons for their support and guidance.

To the Center for Human Appearance at the University of Pennsylvania for their commitment to scholarly activity.

To our Wives, Eileen Quinn and Sarah Granquist, for their tolerance and unwavering encouragement.

About the companion website

Atlas of Temporomandibular Joint Surgery is accompanied by a companion website:

www.wiley.com/go/quinn/atlasTMJsurgery

The website includes:
- Videos showing procedures described in the book
  - Incision design and placement for approaches to the TMJ
  - Stock alloplastic fossa placement
  - Eminoplasty
  - Condylectomy
  - Alloplastic total joint replacement
- Powerpoints of all figures from the book for downloading

CHAPTER 1

Surgical decision making for temporomandibular joint surgery

Correct diagnosis and surgical planning is the key to successful surgical outcomes. Many controversies exist in the management, indications for surgery, and the correct surgical procedure in temporomandibular joint disease. As a number of interventions and management schemes are currently accepted in the literature, these controversies only serve to complicate decision making in temporomandibular joint surgery for internal derangement, trauma, and management of benign and malignant disorders. Several excellent comprehensive textbooks on temporomandibular joint disorders explore the basis for these controversies and provide a historical and scientific overview of this problematic area of maxillofacial surgery.

The intent of this text is simply to illustrate the technical aspects of the various surgical procedures on the temporomandibular joint. No attempt was made to champion a single approach to temporomandibular joint surgery. Ultimately, only well-designed clinical studies can prove, or disprove, the safety and efficacy of the individual procedures. It is our hope that scientific evidence will one day provide the *sine qua non* that will dictate the proper role

for all the potential surgical modalities, including arthroscopy, meniscal repair, and the use of both autogenous and alloplastic materials in joint reconstruction, and eventually, the use of tissue engineering in the management of temporomandibular joint reconstruction. Although serious mistakes have been made in the management of the temporomandibular joint, surgeons cannot allow the failures of the past to obscure the needs of the future.

This text is based on the assumption that primarily extra-articular conditions are most amenable to nonsurgical care. Patients with true internal derangements may benefit from nonsurgical care, and all these modalities should be exhausted before proceeding with any surgical option. The following algorithms are useful as guidelines but must always be modified according to the needs of the individual patient. These algorithms list only current acceptable surgical techniques for various conditions and make no attempt to advocate one surgical procedure over another one. Because several excellent comprehensive texts dealing with arthroscopic techniques are available, this book deals only with open-joint surgical procedures.

Atlas of Temporomandibular Joint Surgery, Second Edition. Edited by Peter D. Quinn and Eric J. Granquist.
© 2015 John Wiley & Sons, Inc. Published 2015 by John Wiley & Sons, Inc.
Companion Website: www.wiley.com/go/quinn/atlasTMJsurgery

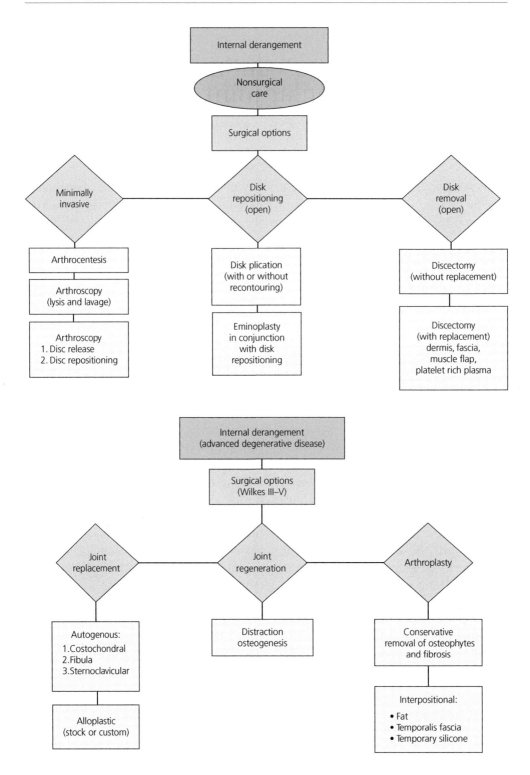

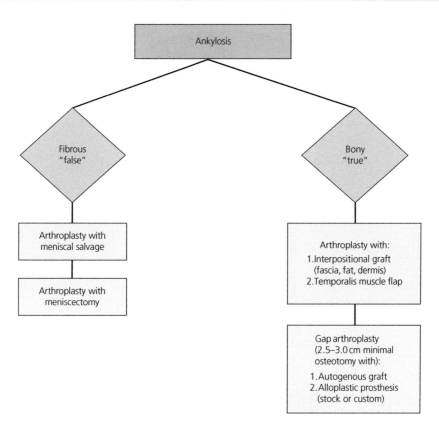

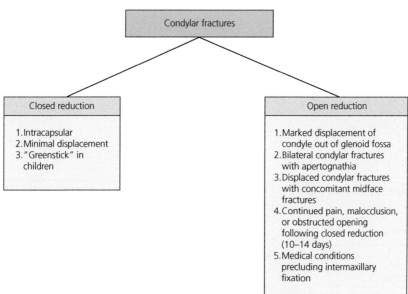

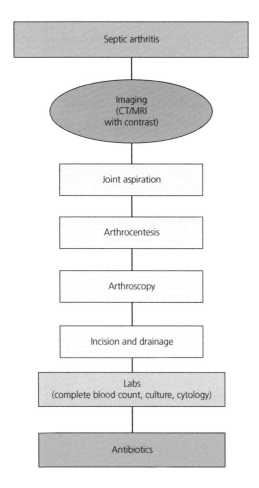

Septic arthritis

Imaging
(CT/MRI
with contrast)

Joint aspiration

Arthrocentesis

Arthroscopy

Incision and drainage

Labs
(complete blood count, culture, cytology)

Antibiotics

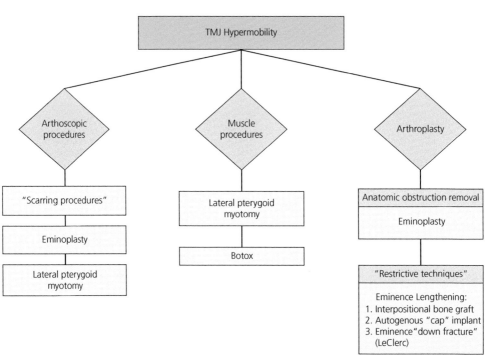

TMJ Hypermobility

Arthoscopic procedures

Muscle procedures

Arthroplasty

"Scarring procedures"

Eminoplasty

Lateral pterygoid myotomy

Lateral pterygoid myotomy

Botox

Anatomic obstruction removal

Eminoplasty

"Restrictive techniques"

Eminence Lengthening:
1. Interpositional bone graft
2. Autogenous "cap" implant
3. Eminence "down fracture" (LeClerc)

CHAPTER 2

Diagnostic imaging of the temporomandibular joint

Because of the anatomic complexity of the temporomandibular joint (TMJ) and its proximity to the base of the skull, temporal bone, mastoid air cells, and auditory structures, imaging of the joint structures can be problematic. Imaging studies should aid the clinician in diagnosis and surgical planning. The choice of imaging modality should be based on history and physical exam. Consideration should be given to the amount of radiation, invasiveness of the exam, ability to obtain the study, and cost. The study that is able to best answer the clinical question while maximizing cost effectiveness should be utilized.

Plain film, tomograms, and orthopantogram radiography

Plain films, tomograms, and orthopantogram (panoramic) studies provide good osseous detail of the TMJ, with minimal radiation, and are easily obtained. As such, they are often an excellent choice for initial evaluation of TMJ pathology.

Standard transcranial (lateral oblique) views provide a global view of bony architecture of the articular surfaces. If possible, a submental vertex film can be taken to allow the lateral oblique transcranial projection to be angled directly through the long access of the condyle. This improves the image quality and also allows standardization of subsequent transcranial views. With the exception of emergency room visits for trauma or dislocation, tomograms or panoramic radiographs have largely replaced these studies.

Tomography has been widely available since the early 1940s and provides finer detail for the examination of osseous abnormalities than detected by plain film techniques. The angle-corrected tomograms for sagittal tomography are recommended so that the sectioning is always perpendicular to the long axis of the condyle. This gives a truer picture of the condyle position, gives the best evaluation of erosion and osteophyte formation, and allows subsequent comparative studies to be performed by use of a standard method. The angle can be determined by measuring the angle between the condylar axis and a horizontal baseline on a submental vertex view.

Orthopantogram radiographs have been described as "curved tomograms." They are, in fact, laminograms of a single

Atlas of Temporomandibular Joint Surgery, Second Edition. Edited by Peter D. Quinn and Eric J. Granquist.
© 2015 John Wiley & Sons, Inc. Published 2015 by John Wiley & Sons, Inc.
Companion Website: www.wiley.com/go/quinn/atlasTMJsurgery

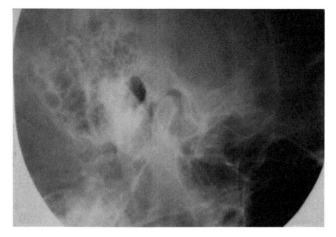

Figure 2.1 Transcranial radiograph, demonstrating the limitations of this study. Note the overlap of adjacent structures with the glenoid fossa and mandibular condyle.

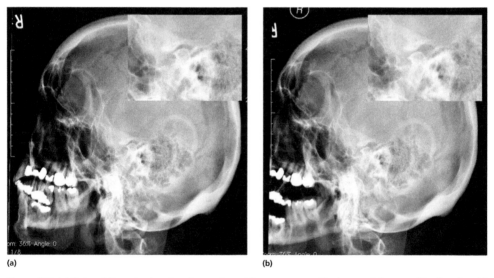

(a)   (b)

Figure 2.2 (a) Later oblique in the closed mouth position, note mandibular condyle seated in the glenoid fossa (inset). (b) Lateral oblique in open mouth position, note translation of TMJ condyle (inset).

plane. This study provides osseous imaging of the condyle and fossa, includes both joints, as well as the entire mandible for comparison of symmetry. Disadvantages include "ghost" images, distortion (~20%), and less detail when compared to angle-corrected condylar tomograms. Newer units allow for separate positioning of right and left joints, creating more correct placement of the condyle in the zone of focus, improving resolution. Some units are able to produce tomograms, allowing increased anatomic detail of the condyle.

Plain films and tomographic images are beneficial in assessing osseous changes in the condyle and eminence. However, the use of these films to assess condylar position with any accuracy is questionable at best. Several studies have shown that the position of the condyle, as depicted in these radiographic techniques, is of little clinical significance. Open- and closed-mouth tomographic views can provide valuable information with regard to condylar translation. Although it has been postulated that during normal range of motion the greatest convexity of the condyle reaches the greatest convexity of the articular eminence, several studies have shown that a majority of patients actually can translate beyond the greatest convexity of the articular eminence without subluxation, dislocation, or any symptoms. These studies can diagnose restricted range of motion but do not provide enough information to determine the etiology of that restriction.

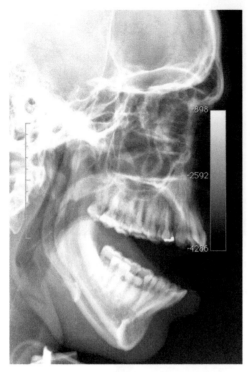

Figure 2.3 Lateral cephalogram showing bilateral dislocation of the temporomandibular joints. Note anteriorly positioned mandible and open bite.

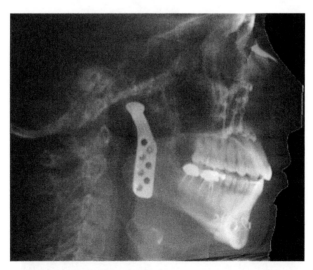

Figure 2.4 Postoperative lateral cephalogram. Study demonstrates good condylar prosthetic position and occlusal relationship.

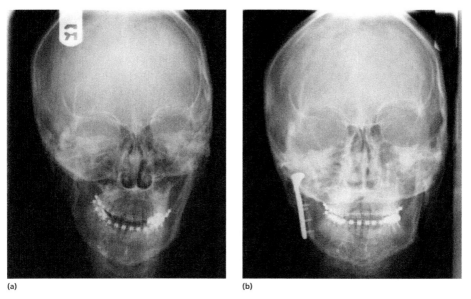

(a)   (b)

Figure 2.5 (a) Preoperative posterior–anterior (PA) skull film. Note facial asymmetry involving the maxilla and mandible. (b) Postoperative PA demonstrating achievement of facial symmetry. Condylar prosthesis is well aligned. Note maxillary hardware from Le Fort I procedure.

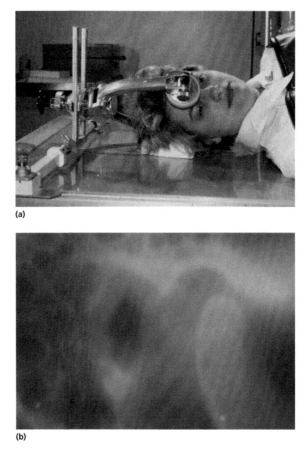

Figure 2.6 (a) Patient positioned for angle-corrected temporomandibular joint tomograms. Source: Quinn 1998, figure 2.3a, p. 7. Reproduced with permission of Elsevier. (b) Angle-corrected tomogram of right temporomandibular joint.

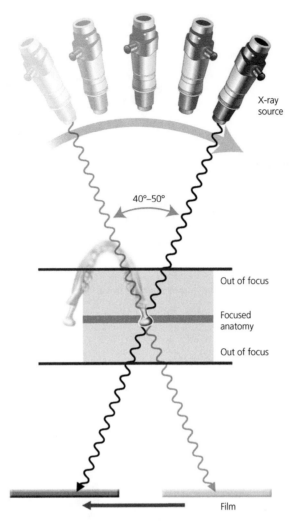

Figure 2.7 Tomographic technique—basic principle of tomographic X-rays. Both the radiation source and film are moving simultaneously to blur all the anatomy anterior and posterior to the point of plane convergence.

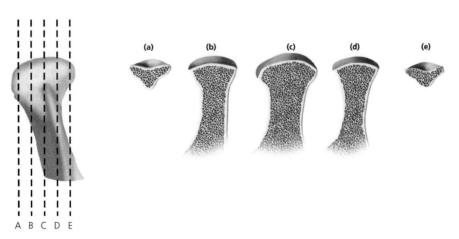

Figure 2.8 Representation of sagittal cuts in standard tomographic condylar films showing anatomy from the most lateral to the most medial cut (a) progressing medial (b, c, d) to the most medial cut (e).

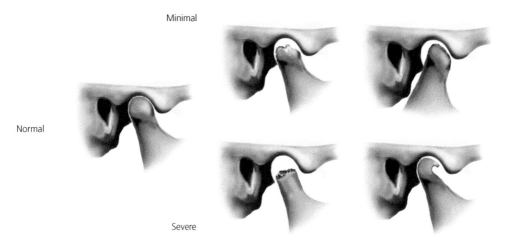

Figure 2.9 Typical contours of lateral condylar tomograms in varying stages of degenerative joint disease.

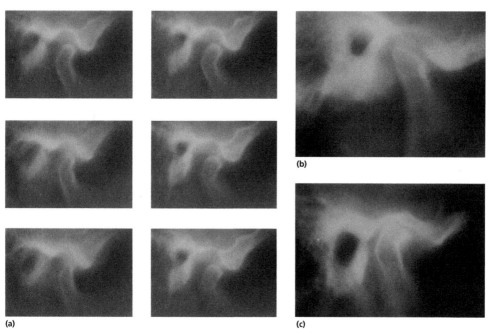

Figure 2.10 (a) Temporomandibular joint-tomographic series depicting excellent osseous detail with 5 mm cuts. (b) Sclerosis and condylar head flatting. (c) "Bird-beaking" of condyle in late stage degeneration.

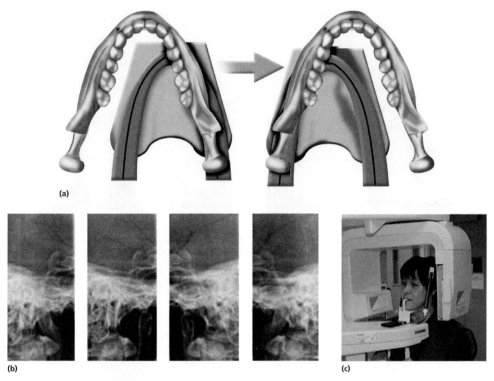

(a)

(b)   (c)

Figure 2.11 (a) Patient positioned for panoramic tomogram of the temporomandibular joints.
(b) Example of programmed condylar views available on most panoramic tomographic units.
(c) Bilateral positioning techniques for specific temporomandibular joint-panoramic X-ray imaging
positioned to align the condyle into the center of the "trough" of resolution of the panoramic
tomogram.

Arthrography

Magnetic resonance imaging (MRI) has replaced arthrography in most instances for soft tissue imaging of the TMJ. Arthrography can offer valuable information not always available through any other imaging technique. It is the only imaging technique that demonstrates perforations in the disk in "real-time" because the operator can see the dye escape from the inferior to the superior joint space during the initial injection. The usual technique involves injection of a water-soluble, iodinated contrast material into the inferior joint space under fluoroscopy. A videotaped arthrofluoroscopic study could clearly show the various stages of disk displacement with or without reduction but is unable to show medial or lateral disk displacement. Potential complications from arthrography include allergic reaction to the contrast material, infection, and pain and swelling secondary to the invasive puncture technique used during the procedure.

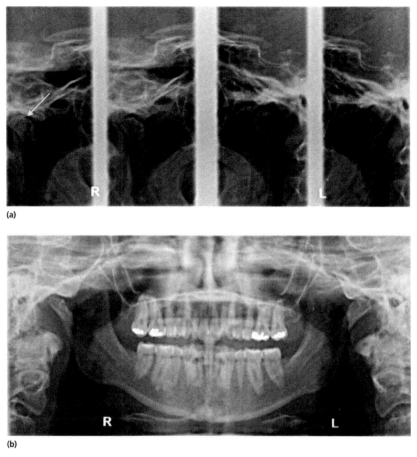

(a)

(b)

Figure 2.12 (a) Dedicated tomogram showing bilateral degenerative joint disease, note the subchondral cyst on the right condyle (arrow). (b) Panorex of same patient. Note improved anatomic detail is evident in the tomogram (a) when compared to the panorex (b).

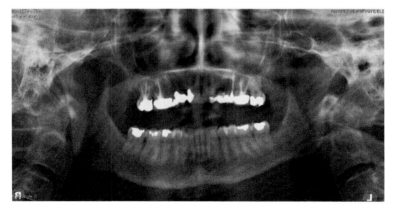

Figure 2.13 Panorex demonstrating left TMJ "bird beaking" and condylar sclerosis.

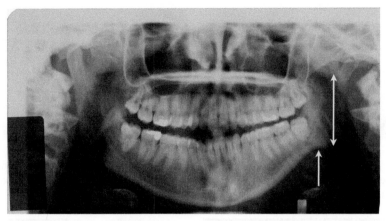

Figure 2.14 Patient with temporomandibular joint osteoarthritis prior to the completion of facial growth. Note decreased ramus height (double arrow) and increased premasseteric (antegonial) notching (single arrow).

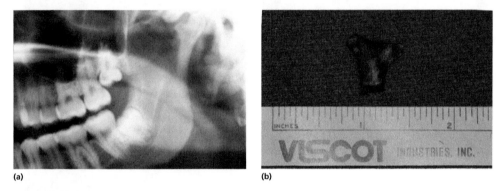

(a)   (b)

Figure 2.15 "Hoof" deformity in condylar head, secondary to condylar trauma during growth. Panorex (a) and status-post resection (b).

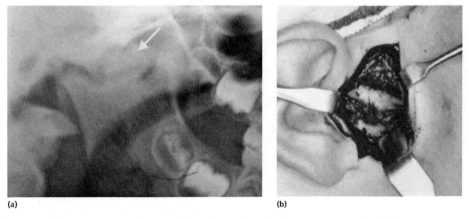

(a)   (b)

Figure 2.16 (a) Panorex of a pediatric patient with ankylosis of the temporomandibular joint. Note displaced condylar head superior to the sigmoid notch (arrow). (b) Intraoperative photo of the same patient showing the ankylosis and fibrous union of the condyle to the skull base.

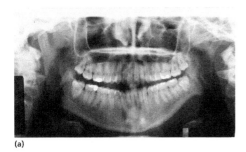
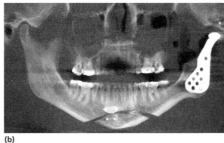

(a) (b)

Figure 2.17 (a) Preoperative panorex of a patient with facial asymmetry secondary to temporomandibular juvenile rheumatoid arthritis. (b) Immediate postoperative panorex following total joint replacement, Le Fort I osteotomy and genioplasty.

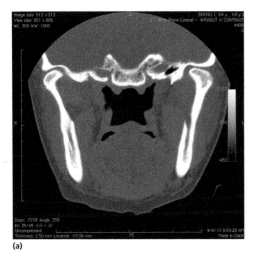

(a)

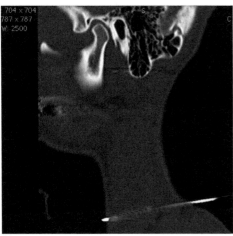

(b)

Figure 2.18 (a) Coronal computer-tomography (CT) in bone windows, showing normal temporomandibular joints. (b) Sagittal CT in bone windows, showing a normal temporomandibular joint.

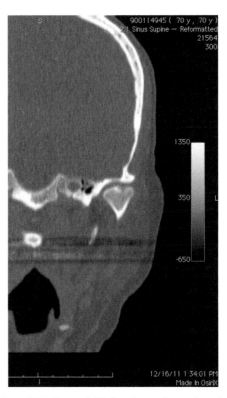

Figure 2.19 Coronal CT showing early erosion of the left condyle in a patient with osteoarthritis.

Computer tomography, 3D reconstruction, and computer planning

Computer tomography (CT) of the TMJ is currently the best method for assessing bony pathologic conditions of the TMJ and allows assessment of the proximity of

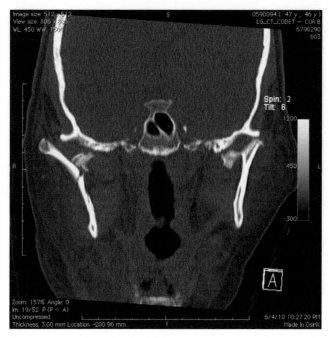

Figure 2.20 Coronal CT showing bilateral sagittal fractures of the condylar heads and a right subcondylar fracture with severe lateral displacement.

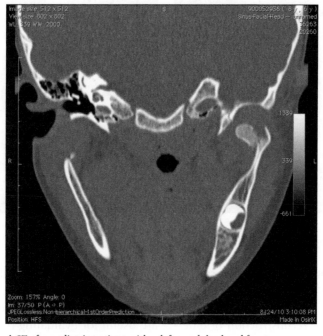

Figure 2.21 Coronal CT of a pediatric patient with a left condylar head fracture.

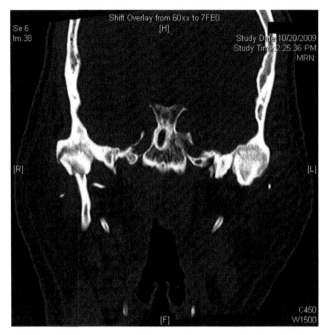

Figure 2.22 Coronal CT demonstrating bilateral TMJ ankylosis.

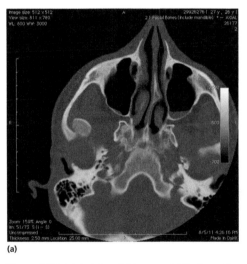

(a)

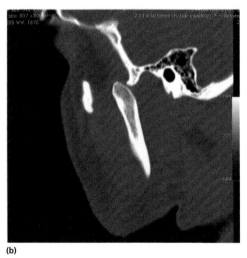

(b)

Figure 2.23 (a) Axial and (b) coronal CT of a patient with right dislocated condyle.

surrounding vital structures for surgical planning. Most modern scanners are able to produce fine cuts of the area of interest, which allows for reconstruction of different views (e.g., axial, coronal, sagittal) and renders patient positioning less crucial.

Sagittal views are excellent at evaluating the condylar anatomy, glenoid fossa, and articular eminence. Coronal images are useful for evaluating trauma for condylar displacement. Soft tissue windows may be useful when treating tumors

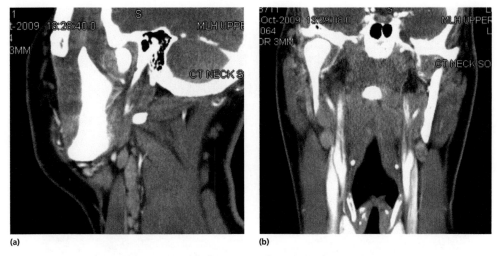

Figure 2.24 (a) Axial and (b) coronal CT soft tissue windows with contrast of patient with septic arthritis. Note rim enhancing of the contrast around the temporomandibular joint and anterior displacement of the condyle.

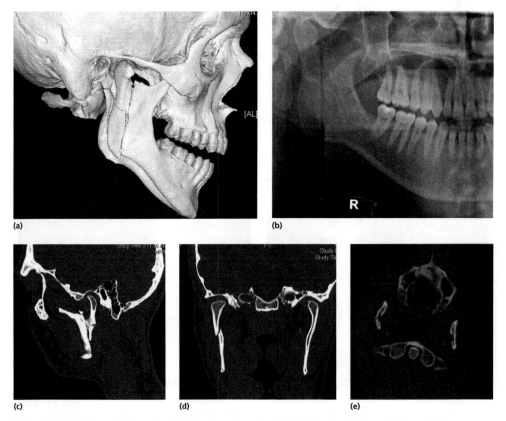

Figure 2.25 (a) 3D reconstruction, (b) panorex (c), sagittal CT, (d) coronal CT, and (e) axial CT of a patient with a comminuted fracture involving the ramus and subcondylar region. Note how the 3D reconstruction aids in demonstrating the relation of the fracture.

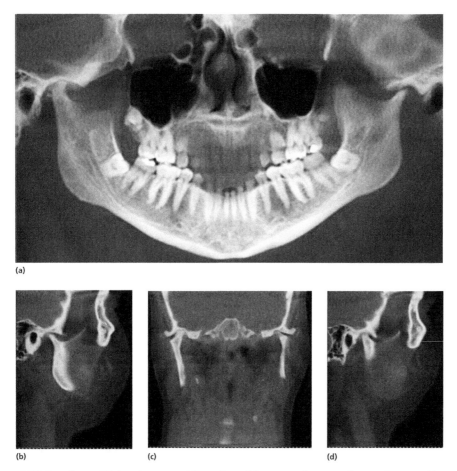

(a)

(b)   (c)   (d)

Figure 2.26 Cone beam CT showing severe bilateral condylar resorption secondary to rheumatoid arthritis. (a) Panorex from cone beam CT. (b) Right sagittal cone beam CT. (c) Coronal cone beam CT. (d) Left sagittal cone beam CT.

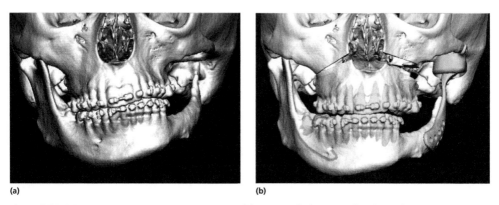

(a)   (b)

Figure 2.27 (a) Preoperative 3D reconstruction used for surgical planning. (b) Planned 3D surgical reconstruction with the maxilla and mandible repositioned into the desired position, allowing for the design of the custom TMJ prosthesis.

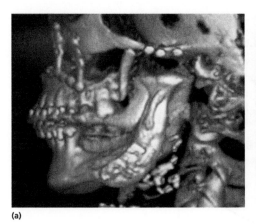
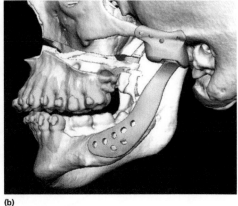

(a)   (b)

Figure 2.28 (a) Postoperative 3D reconstruction using cone beam CT. (b) Preoperative planned position. Note artifact from cobalt-chrome prosthesis.

involving the TMJ, but in most cases, evaluation of the soft tissue anatomy of the joint with a CT study is difficult. Finally, CT scans with contrast are invaluable when evaluating a patient with suspect septic arthritis, as these studies are readily available to most practitioners.

Three-dimensional CT images can be helpful in case of gross asymmetry for orthognathic surgery or joint reconstruction planning. Also, these imaging studies can be utilized in panfacial fractures involving the TMJ. Planning software is available to evaluate treatment prior to surgery. Surgical navigation can also be utilized with CT scans to ensure surgical osteotomies are placed correctly.

Magnetic resonance imaging

Magnetic resonance (MR) images can be obtained in the sagittal, axial, and coronal planes. Thinner sections result in improved image quality because "volume averaging" of the structures is reduced. In most normal scanning sequences, both T1 weighted and T2 weighted images will be obtained. With the most commonly used pulsed sequence (spin-echo), T1 weighted images highlight fat within the tissues and T2 weighted images may give a poorer image quality but highlight water-containing structures. These T2 weighted images are particularly helpful when the operator is attempting to determine whether a joint effusion exists. If concern for effusion exists, particularly for patients with rheumatologic arthritis or infection, an MRI with contrast should be obtained. Dynamic MRI is available to assess joint function, though is not widely used in clinical practice.

The major contraindication to MRI is posed by ferromagnetic metals. Ferromagnetic clips used to treat a cerebral aneurysm are an absolute contraindication to MR scanning. The other absolute contraindication occurs with patients who have cardiac pacemakers. Non-ferromagnetic metals, such as those used in orthodontic braces, cobalt chromium prostheses, and titanium implants do not pose problems related to magnetic fields but do compromise image quality because of artifact production.

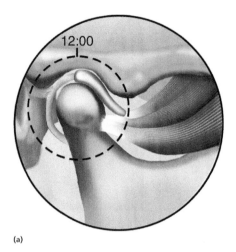

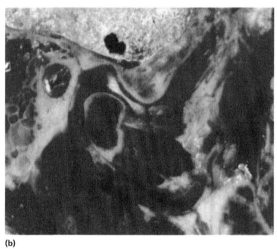

Figure 2.29 Diagrammatic representation showing normal condyle disk position with junction of posterior attachment and posterior band of disk aligned approximately at the 12 o'clock position with regard to the condylar surface (a) and sagittal cadaver demonstrating normal condylar-disk position (b).

Although MRI is clearly preferred for assessing internal derangements, all patients with joint symptoms do not require MR studies. Tomograms or condyle-specific panoramic films are certainly adequate to assess whether a patient has gross degenerative changes within the joint. Clinical exam and history are used to diagnose disk displacement with and without reduction. If a reasonable attempt at conservative therapy does not improve symptoms and further documentation of the internal derangement is necessary to determine whether the patient may be a surgical candidate, then MRI should be considered. MRI is also useful when evaluating medial and lateral disk herniation.

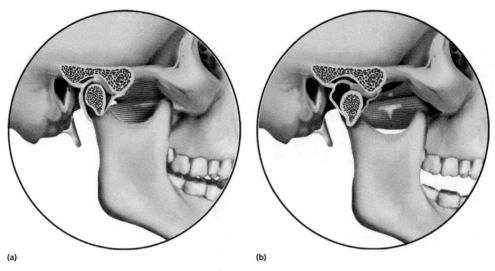

(a)   **(b)**

Figure 2.30 Normal closed (a) and open condyle and disk position (b).

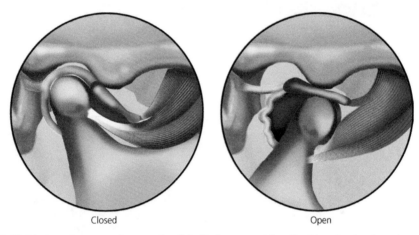

Closed   Open

Figure 2.31 Diagram demonstrating anterior disk displacement (closed) with reduction (open).

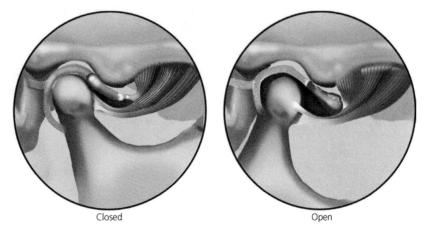

Closed   Open

Figure 2.32 Diagram demonstrating anteriorly displaced disk (closed) without reduction (open). Notice decreased translation movement of the condylar head.

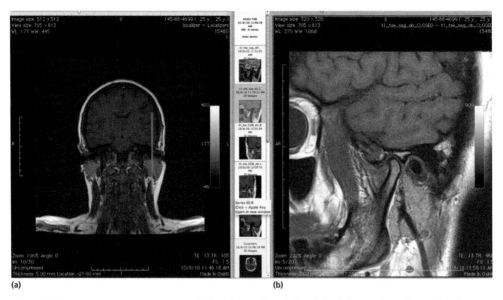

(a) (b)

Figure 2.33 (a) Locator image. (b) Normal closed mouth T1 MRI of the left TMJ (as indicated by the image in (a)).

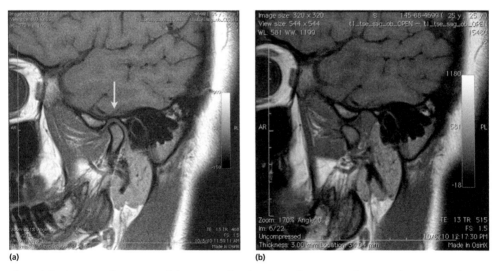

(a) (b)

Figure 2.34 (a) Normal T1 image of the TMJ in the closed mouth position. (b) Normal T1 MRI in the open mouth position.

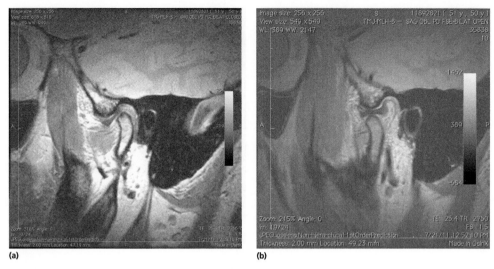

(a)   (b)

Figure 2.35 (a, b) Open and closed views of right temporomandibular joint with early anterior disk displacement with reduction.

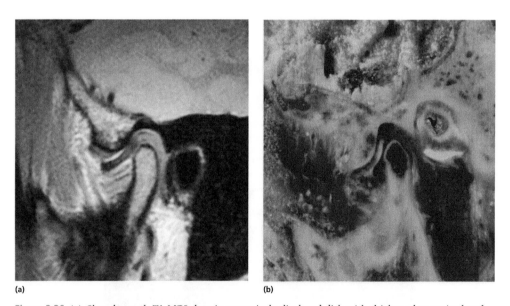

(a)   (b)

Figure 2.36 (a) Closed mouth T1 MRI showing anteriorly displaced disk with thickened posterior band. Note minimal osseous changes. (b) Cryosection showing early pathologic changes with anterior disk displacement. Note thickening of retrodiscal tissue.

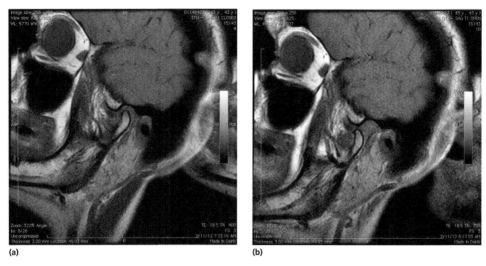

(a)   (b)

Figure 2.37 Open (a) and closed (b) MR image of right temporomandibular joint showing anterior disk displacement without reduction.

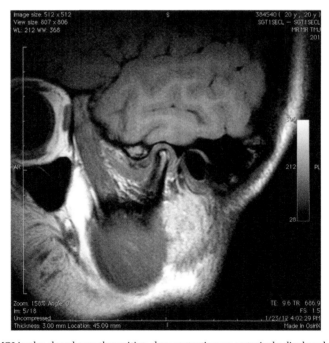

Figure 2.38 T1 MRI in the closed mouth position demonstrating an anteriorly displaced disk with disk deformity.

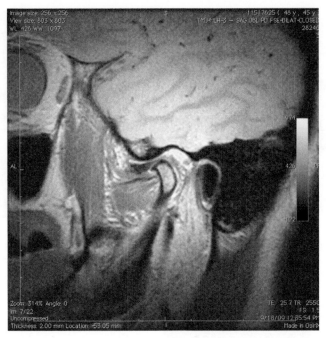

Figure 2.39 T1 MRI in the open-mouth position showing an anteriorly displaced disk without reduction and "bird beaking" of the mandibular condyle. Loss of disk anatomy seen here is indicative of long-standing displacement and with loss of the normal disk biconcavity.

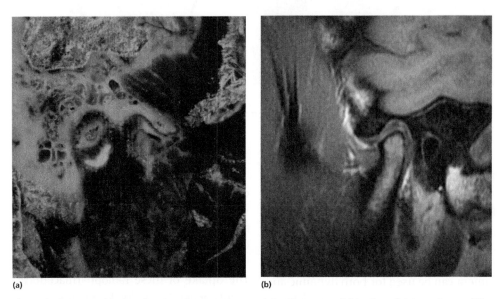

(a)   (b)

Figure 2.40 (a) Cryosection showing degenerative condylar changes and thinning of the meniscus with loss of the normal 3-1-2 disk dimension (anterior band 3mm: intermediate zone 1 mm: posterior band 2 mm). (b) MRI T1 demonstrating similar findings.

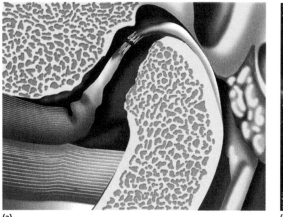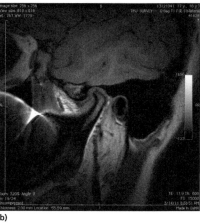

(a) (b)

Figure 2.41 (a) Diagram showing advanced degenerative joint disease. (b) MRI showing anteriorly displaced disk with condylar degeneration, disk thinning, and posterior band thickening.

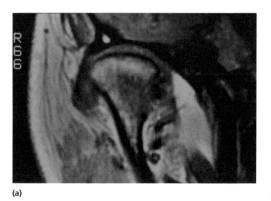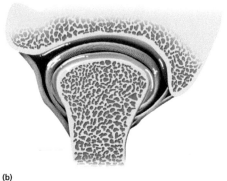

(a) (b)

Figure 2.42 (a) Coronal MRI showing lateral disk herniation. (b) Diagram demonstrating normal disk and capsule attachments.

Bone scans

Radionucleotide imaging of the TMJ can provide information about the dynamics of bone and soft tissue metabolism in a variety of pathologic states. A scintillation camera can be used for both dynamic and static imaging in which a gamma detector quantifies gamma ray emissions from injected isotopes such as technetium 99.

These technetium-labeled phosphate complexes are given to patients by intravenous injection, and then the patients are studied in a phased technique with images performed immediately after injection and at several delayed intervals. The uptake of these radiopharmaceutical agents depends on blood flow to the TMJ structures. Uptake in the TMJ is affected by inflammation, bone remodeling, and

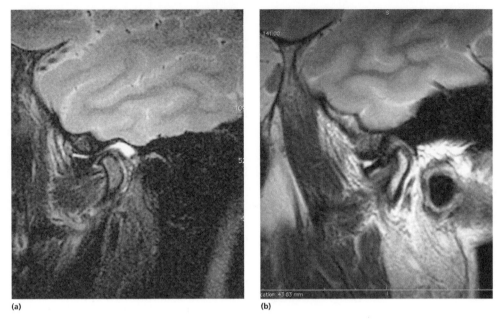

Figure 2.43 (a) T2 MRI with contrast demonstration anterior joint space effusion and enhancement of the retrodiskal tissue. (b) T2 MRI with contrast demonstrating superior joint space effusion.

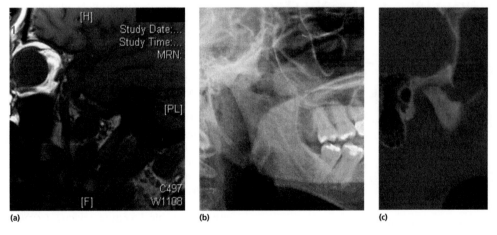

Figure 2.44 (a) MRI, (b) panorex, and (c) cone beam CT of a patient with TMJ ankylosis.

osteoblastic activity. Higher activity is seen at sites of growth, inflammation, and neoplasia and areas where reactive bone is formed during reparative processes. Because they are rather nonspecific, radionucleotide images can be difficult to interpret without good clinical correlation. Radionucleotide images can be helpful in cases such as occult osteomyelitis and condylar hyperplasia (Figure 2.45).

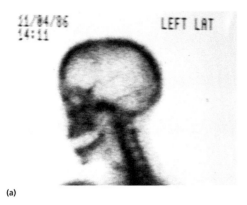

(a)

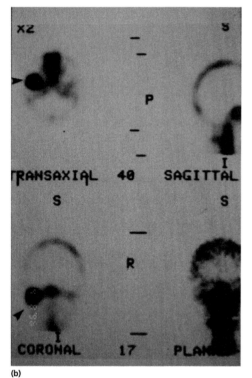

(b)

Figure 2.45 Technetium 99 bone scan.
(a) Nonspecific positive bone scan of left
temporomandibular joint, secondary to
psoriatic arthritis. (b) Positive bone scan
with enhancement of the right
temporomandibular joint secondary to
condylar hyperplasia.

Further reading

Brand JW. *et al.* (1989) The effects of temporomandibular joint internal derangement and
degenerative joint disease on tomographic
and arthrotomographie images. *Oral Surg Oral
Med Oral Pathol*, 67:220.

Bronstein SL. *et al.* (1981) Internal derangements of the temporomandibular joint: correlation of arthrographic with surgical findings.
J Oral Surg, 39:572.

Eckerdal O. (1973) Tomography of the temporomandibular joint: correlation between
tomographic image and histologic sections in
a three-dimensional system. *Acta Radiol Suppl*,
329(suppl):196.

Gray RJM. *et al.* (1990) Histopathological and
scintigraphic features of condylar hyperplasia.
Int J Oral Maxillofac Surg, 19:65.

Habets LL. *et al.* (1987) The orthopantomogram:
an aid in diagnosis of temporomandibular
joint problems. I. The factor of vertical magni-
fication. *J Oral Rehabil*, 14:475.

Helms CA. *et al.* (1982) Computed tomography of
the meniscus of the temporomandibular joints:
preliminary observations. *Radiology*, 145:719.

Hussain AM. *et al.* (2008) Role of different
imaging modalities in assessment of temporomandibular joint erosions and osteophytes:
a systemic review. *Dentomaxillofac Radiol*, 37:63.

Kaplan PA. *et al.* (1986) Inferior joint space
arthrography of normal temporomandibular
joints: reassessment of diagnostic criteria.
Radiology, 159:585.

Katzberg RW, Westesson P-L. (1993) *Diagnosis
of the temporomandibular joint*, WB Saunders,
Philadelphia.

Koh K-J. *et al.* (2009) Relationship between
clinical and magnetic resonance imaging
diagnosis and findings in degenerative and
inflammatory temporomandibular joint disease: a systemic literature review. *J Orofac
Pain*, 23:123.

Kurita K. *et al.* (1992) Temporomandibular
joint: diagnosis of medial and lateral disk displacement with anteroposterior arthrography: correlation with cryosections. *Oral Surg
Oral Med Oral Pathol*, 73:364.

Manzione JV. *et al.* (1984) Internal derangements
of the temporomandibular joint: diagnosis by

direct sagittal computed tomography. *Radiology*, 150:111.

Matteson SR. *et al.* (1985) Bone scanning with technetium phosphate to assess condylar hyperplasia. *Oral Surg Oral Med Oral Pathol*, 60:356.

Petersson A. (1991) Plain film imaging and tomography. In *Images of the temporomandibular joint: Cranio Clinics International*. (Eds P-L Westesson and RW Katzberg). Williams and Wilkins, Baltimore.

Pullinger AG. *et al.* (1986) Tomographic analysis of mandibular condyle position in diagnostic subgroups of temporomandibular disorders. *J Prosthet Dent*, 55:723.

Ribeiro-Rotta RF. *et al.* (2011) Do computed tomography and magnetic resonance imaging add to temporomandibular joint disorders? A systematic review of diagnostic efficacy. *J Oral Rehabil*, 38:120.

Sano T. *et al.* (2004) Common abnormalities in temporomandibular joint imaging. *Curr Probl Diagn Radiol*, 33:16.

Schellhas KP, Wilkes CH. (1989) Temporomandibular joint inflammation: comparison of MR to fast scanning with T1 and T2 weighted imaging techniques. *AJR Am J Roentgenol*, 153:93.

Schellhas KP. *et al.* (1987) Temporomandibular joint: MR imaging of internal derangements and postoperative changes. *AJR Am J Roentgenol*, 8:1093.

Simon DC. *et al.* (1985) Direct sagittal CT of the temporomandibular joint. *Radiology*, 157:545.

Thompson JR. *et al.* (1984) Temporomandibular joints: high resolution computed tomographic evaluation. *Radiology*, 150:105.

Westesson P-L, Brooks SL. (1992) Temporomandibular joint: magnetic resonance evidence of joint effusion relative to joint pain and internal derangement. *AJR*, 159:559.

Westesson P-L. *et al.* (1978) Temporomandibular joint: comparison of MR images with cryosectional anatomy. *Radiology*, 164:645.

Westesson P-L. *et al.* (1986) Temporomandibular joint: correlation between single-contrast video arthrography and post-modern morphology. *Radiology*, 160:767.

CHAPTER 3

Surgical approaches to the temporomandibular joint

Serious morbidity from facial nerve injury, scar formation, or ear injury can overshadow the mechanical improvements in joint function and the amelioration of painful symptoms. Incisions were described by Humphrey in 1856 for condylectomy, Ricdel for meniscectomy in 1883, and Annandale for disk repositioning in 1887. The main potential anatomic problems in temporomandibular joint surgery are the facial nerve and the terminal branches of the external carotid artery. Approaches to the joint include the following: preauricular, endaural, postauricular, rhytidectomy, retromandibular, and intraoral. Ideally, the selected approach should accomplish the following: maximize exposure for the specific procedure; avoid damage to the branches of the facial nerve, major vessels (e.g., internal maxillary artery and retromandibular vein), parotid gland, and ear; and maximize use of natural skin creases for cosmetic wound closure.

Applied anatomy

Facial nerve

The main trunk of the facial nerve exits from the skull at the stylomastoid foramen. The suture line between the tympanic and mastoid portions of the mastoid bone is a reliable anatomic landmark because the main trunk of the facial nerve lies 6–8 mm inferior and anterior to this tympanomastoid suture. Approximately 1.3 cm of the facial nerve is visible until it divides into temporofacial and cervicofacial branches. In the classic article by Al-Kayat and Bramley (1980), the distance from the lowest point of the external bony auditory canal to the bifurcation was found to be 1.5–2.8 cm (mean, 2.3 cm), and the distance from the postglenoid tubercle to the bifurcation was 2.4–3.5 cm (mean, 3.0 cm). The most variable measurement was the point at which the upper trunk crosses the zygomatic arch. It ranged from 8 to 35 mm anterior to the most anterior portion of the bony external auditory canal (mean, 2.0 cm). By incising the superficial layer of the temporalis fascia and the periosteum over the arch inside the 8 mm boundary, surgeons can prevent damage to the branches of the upper trunk. The temporal branch of the facial nerve emerges from the parotid gland and crosses the zygoma under the temporoparietal fascial to innervate the frontalis muscle ("corrugator muscle") in

Atlas of Temporomandibular Joint Surgery, Second Edition. Edited by Peter D. Quinn and Eric J. Granquist.
© 2015 John Wiley & Sons, Inc. Published 2015 by John Wiley & Sons, Inc.
Companion Website: www.wiley.com/go/quinn/atlasTMJsurgery

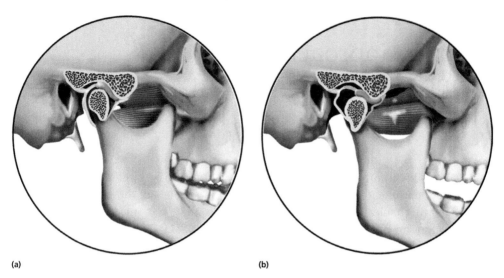

(a)   (b)

Figure 3.1 (a) Normal condyle and fossa with mandible closed. Note the position of the disk, with the posterior aspect at the height of the condyle. (b) Mandible open. Condyle has both rotated and translated along the articular eminence. Note disk has moved anteriorly along with the condyle.

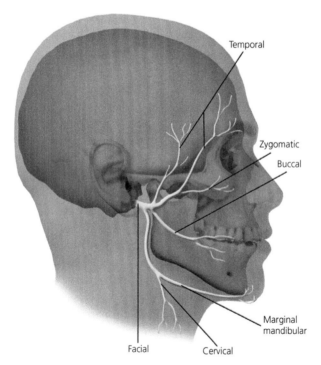

Figure 3.2 Facial nerve emerging from stylomastoid foramen showing division into upper trunk with temporal and zygomatic branches and lower trunk with buccal, marginal mandibular, and cervical branches.

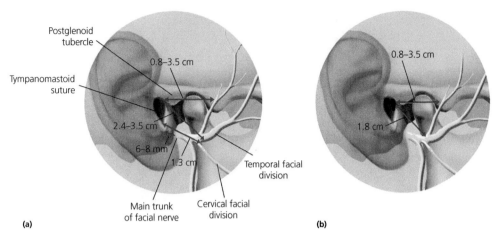

Figure 3.3 (a) Surgical landmarks for identifying the location of main trunk of the facial nerve and the temporal-facial division during temporomandibular arthroplastic dissection. (b) Note the variability at the point where the upper trunk of the facial nerve crosses the zygomatic arch deep to the temporoparietal fascial. The nerve can cross the zygomatic arch from 0.8 to 3.5 cm anterior to the bony auditory canal. Consequently, the plane of dissection must be deep to the temporoparietal fascial as the tissues are retracted anteriorly to gain access to the joint capsule.

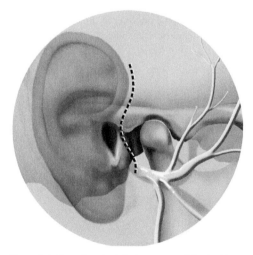

Figure 3.4 Note that the inferior extent of the incision is the soft tissue attachment of the lobule of the ear. Also, the superior arm of the incision can be extended into the temporal hairline at a 45° angle if greater retraction of the surgical flap is necessary.

the forehead. Postsurgical palsy manifests as an inability to raise the eyebrow and ptosis of the brow. Damage to the

zygomatic branch results in temporary or permanent paralysis to the orbicularis oculi and may require temporary patching of the eye to prevent corneal desiccation and abrasion. Permanent nerve damage may necessitate tarsorrhaphy before a more permanent functional approach, such as implantation of a gold weight for gravity-assisted closure of the upper lid, can be used. Galvanic stimulation can be helpful in speeding recovery after a neuropraxia type of injury.

Trigeminal nerve

The auriculotemporal nerve is the first branch of the third division of the trigeminal nerve after it exits the foramen ovale. The auriculotemporal nerve courses from a medial to a lateral direction behind the neck of the condyle and supplies sensation to the skin in the temporal and preauricular region, the anterior external meatus,

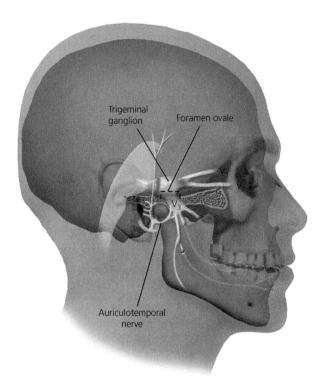

Figure 3.5 Depiction of the auriculotemporal nerve emerging from the third division of the trigeminal nerve coursing behind the neck of the condyle. The nerve innervates the majority of the capsule and meniscal-attachment tissues. The capsule is also innervated by the masseteric and posterior deep temporal nerves.

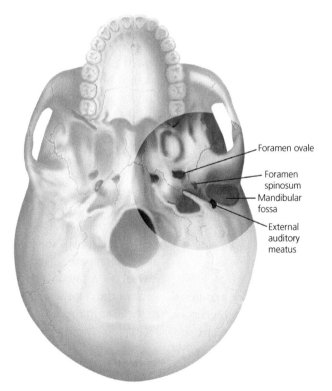

Figure 3.6 Base of skull showing position of foramen ovale in relation to the mandibular fossa. The main trunk of the facial nerve would rarely be encountered during the open joint surgery.

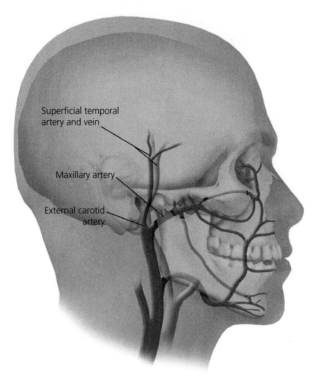

Figure 3.7 Superficial temporal artery and vein, which run just below the subcutaneous tissue anterior to the tragal cartilage.

and the tympanic membrane. Some damage is inevitable during standard joint approaches but rarely poses a problem. The auriculotemporal nerve provides most of the innervation to the capsule of the temporomandibular joint itself. The anterior portion of the joint also receives innervation from the masseteric nerve and the posterior deep temporal nerve. The articular cartilage on the surface of the condyle and the glenoid fossa and the avascular meniscus itself have no innervation. The inferior alveolar branch of the trigeminal nerve enters the mandibular ramus on the medial surface and runs inferiorly and anteriorly until it exits through the mental foramen. This nerve innervates the teeth, anterior gingiva, and lip. Radiographic assessment of the exact course of this nerve through the mandible is necessary if screws will be placed through the ramus as is necessary for prosthetic joint replacement.

Vascular anatomy

The external carotid artery terminates in two branches: the superficial temporal and internal maxillary arteries. The superficial temporal artery and vein are routinely ligated during preauricular approaches, and the internal maxillary is usually not encountered unless a condylectomy is performed. If a condylectomy is performed, great care should be taken to protect deep soft tissue structures with the aid of the Dunn-Dautrey retractors as the internal maxillary artery normally runs-approximately 3 mm medial from the midsigmoid notch. The most commonly

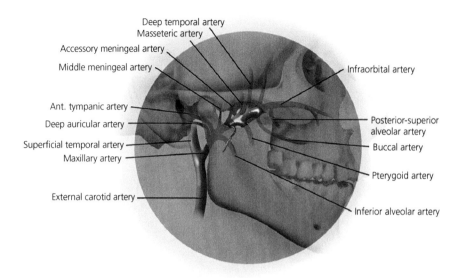

Figure 3.8 Detailed view of the maxillary artery and its branches. The middle meningeal artery courses medially from the maxillary artery, and the masseteric artery runs laterally through the sigmoid notch. Both the maxillary and masseteric arteries can be damaged during extensive dissection.

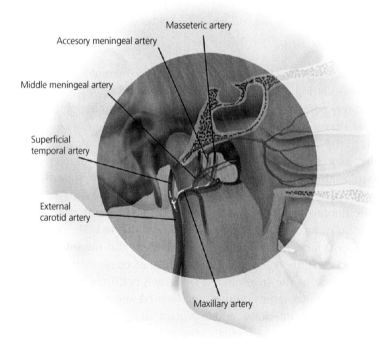

Figure 3.9 View from medial aspect of the mandible. Note proximity of middle meningeal, external maxillary, and masseteric arteries. Care should be taken to protect these structures at the level of the condylar neck and sigmoid notch during osteotomies.

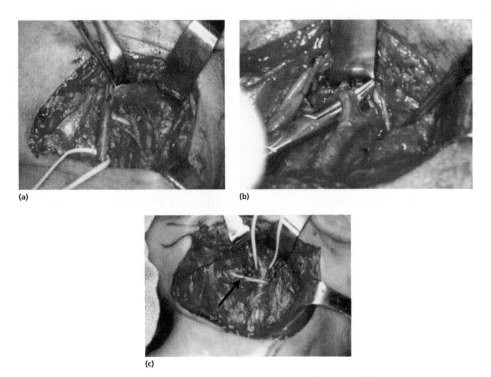

Figure 3.10 (a) Isolation of the external carotid artery. (b) Note confirmation of branches off the external carotid artery to distinguish it from the internal carotid artery. (c) Hypoglossal nerve overlying the carotid sheath (black arrow).

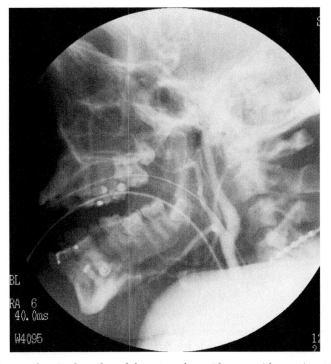

Figure 3.11 Angiogram showing branches of the external carotid artery with prominent facial and internal maxillary branches.

injured artery during temporomandibular procedures is the middle meningeal artery. Pogrel, in a cadaver study of structures medial to the temporomandibular joint, found the middle meningeal artery to be a mean of 31 mm (range 21–43 mm) medial to the zygomatic arch and a mean of 2.4 mm (range −2 to 8 mm) anterior from the height of the glenoid fossa.

Surgical approaches

Preauricular

The shape of the incision is that of an inverted hockey stick, which follows the natural crease in front of the tragus. This should suffice for most arthroplastic procedures, but if greater access is required, the Al-Kayat and Bramley (1980) modification with temporal extension can be used. An incision is made through skin and subcutaneous tissue to the superficial temporal fascia. The superficial temporal artery and vein run just above the surface of the fascial layer, and the branches of the facial nerve run deep to it, just above the periosteum over the zygomatic arch. Above the zygomatic arch, the superficial layer of the temporal fascia is incised in an oblique line running from the tragus to the superior end of the skin incision. This incision is parallel to the inverted hockey-stick incision. A mosquito hemostat is used to dissect bluntly along the external auditory canal in an anterior-medial direction to the level of the temporomandibular joint capsule. A #15 blade is used to make an incision along the root

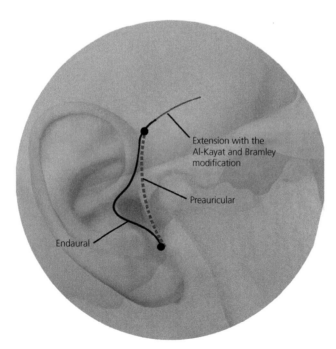

Figure 3.12 Placement of endaural and preauricular incisions. Note the optional temporal extension (Al-Kayat and Bramley modification) for more anterior flap retraction.

of the zygoma through the superficial temporal fascia and the periosteum. This is contiguous with the incision superior to the arch. With blunt hemostat dissection a plane is developed through this incision, just above the white, glistening temporomandibular joint capsule. The incision continues in a skin crease several millimeters anterior to the tragus parallel to the auricle. The incision is carried through the superficial muscular aponeurotic system. This allows dissection to continue along the zygomatic arch, in a safe subperiosteal plane. The dissection can continue anteriorly, exposing the entire temporomandibular joint. The joint can then be safely entered by first injecting 1 cc of lidocaine, insufflating the joint space. This increases the space between the disk, and glenoid fossa, allowing safe entry of a #15 blade at a 45° angle.

Endaural

The endaural incision is simply a cosmetic modification of the standard preauricular approach. Based on a rhytidectomy incision, it moves the skin

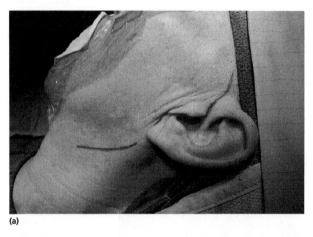

(a)

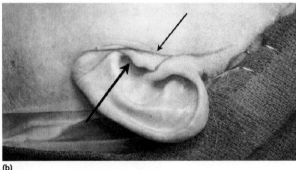

(b)

Figure 3.13 (a) Placement of modified retromandibular approach and endaural incisions. Note well hidden incision placement along the tragus. (b) Comparison of preauricular (thin arrow) and endaural incisions (thick arrow). The endaural incision allows for stepped tissue dissection for improved tissue coverage of the temporomandibular joint.

incision from the pretragal crease posteriorly so that the incision is placed behind the prominence of the tragus itself. Care must be taken not to incise the tragal cartilage because a perichondritis or poor wound healing may result. Once the skin flap is dissected off the tragus, the dissection continues in the same manner as the preauricular approach.

Postauricular

Walters and Geist (1983) popularized a modified postauricular approach to the temporomandibular joint. Although rarely used, the approach has the advantages of excellent exposure of the entire joint and the ability to camouflage the scar in patients who have a tendency to form keloids. The main disadvantage is auricular stenosis, and the approach should not be used in the presence of joint infection or chronic otitis externa. The incision is placed 3–4 mm posterior to the auricular flexure and extended toward the mastoid fascia. Staying above the mastoid fascia (which is contiguous with the temporalis fascia), the incision exposes the superior and posterior circumference of the external auditory canal. Blunt dissection below the external auditory canal creates a plane running anteriorly to separate the pinna. A #10 blade is then used to transect the external auditory canal and retract the ear anteriorly. Dissection can then be carried out through the superficial temporalis fascia and periosteum at the root of the zygoma as previously described. Once the joint surgery is completed, a resorbable 4-0 running

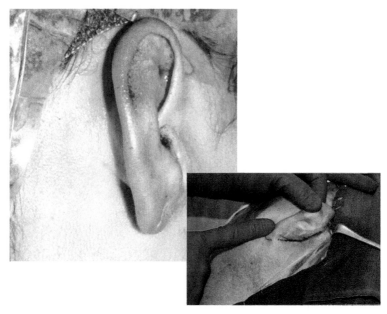

Figure 3.14 Postauricular approach to the temporomandibular joint.

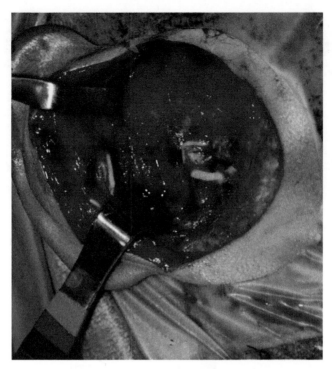

Figure 3.15 Postauricular approach to the temporomandibular joint. The incision has been made through skin and subcutaneous tissue. The external auditory canal has been completely transected. A purse-string sutre has been placed into the transected external auditory canal to prevent hemorrhage into the canal. Although this approach provides excellent visibility, the closure of the external canal can be problematic and auricular stenosis can occur.

suture is used to close the skin of the ear canal only. No attempt is made to suture the cartilage itself.

Rhytidectomy

Major tumor resections may require more extensive joint exposure, and several authors have reported on the use of the rhytidectomy incision. The endaural incision is extended in a curvilinear fashion around the mastoid tip, with an S-shaped extension ending in a submandibular incision. This allows access to the entire posterior border of the mandible and allows for identification of the main trunk of the facial nerve.

Retromandibular

For additional access to the temporomandibular joint for open fracture reduction, costochondral grafting, total alloplastic joint reconstruction, or tumor resection, a submandibular approach is necessary. When combining both incisions, the surgeon must leave an intervening bridge of tissue that extends inferiorly at least 3 cm from the lowest point of the bony external auditory canal. The classic

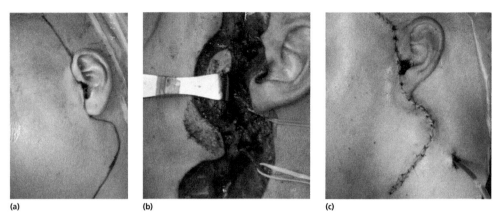

(a)   (b)   (c)

Figure 3.16 (a) Combination of parotidectomy and extended preauricular incision with temporal extension. (b) Auditory alarm connected to terminal branches of the facial nerve. (c) Incision following closure with Jackson–Pratt drain in place.

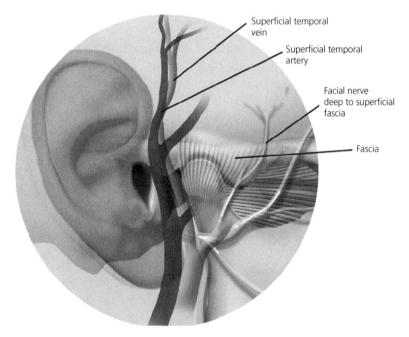

Figure 3.17 Relative position of the superficial temporal artery and vein and the temporal branch of the facial nerve. The vessels are superior to the superficial temporal fascia and the nerve is deep to the fascia.

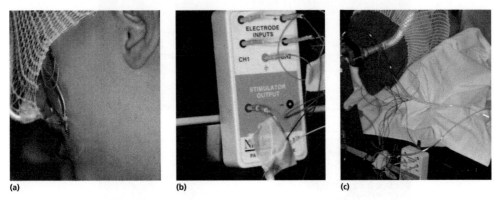

(a)   (b)   (c)

Figure 3.18 (a) Facial nerve monitoring used to identify the frontal and zygomatic branches of the facial nerve. This device is not routinely used for surgical approaches to the temporomandibular joint. It is often useful when the normal anatomic position of the nerve has been altered secondary to pathology or scarring from previous surgeries. (b) An auditory alarm. The electrodes are placed into the monitor and are the terminal branches of the facial nerve. (c) Any direct pressure during surgery will result in an auditory alarm warning the surgeon of their proximity to the facial nerve.

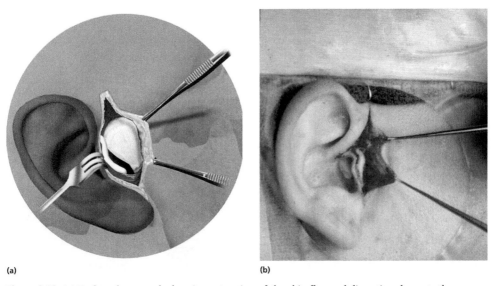

(a)   (b)

Figure 3.19 (a) Endaural approach showing retraction of the skin flap and dissection down to the zygomatic arch. (b) Retraction of the skin flap showing the tragal cartilage.

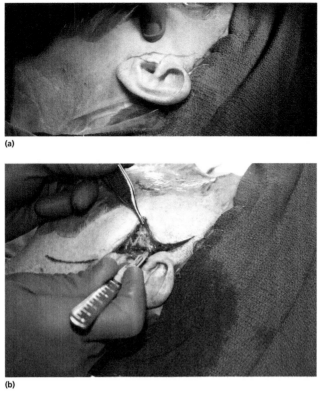

(a)

(b)

Figure 3.20 (a) Comparison of endaural and preauricular approaches. Note position of thumb used to retract the tragus during the endaural incision. (b) Dissection of the skin flap from the tragus during the endaural approach. A small amount of tissue/fat should be left covering the tragal cartilage.

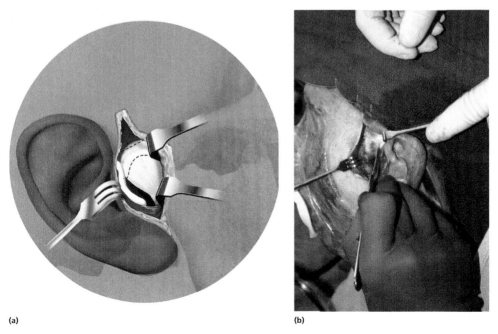

(a)   (b)

Figure 3.21 (a) Retraction of skin flap. (b) Incision through temporoparietal fascial and temporal periosteum.

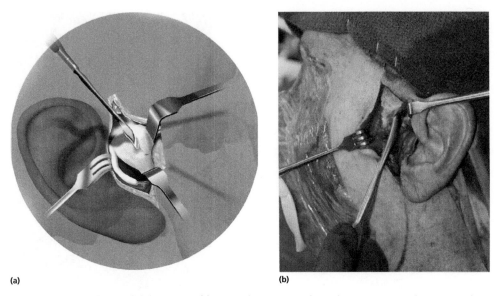

Figure 3.22 (a and b) Careful dissection of fascia and periosteum from the zygomatic arch exposing the joint capsule.

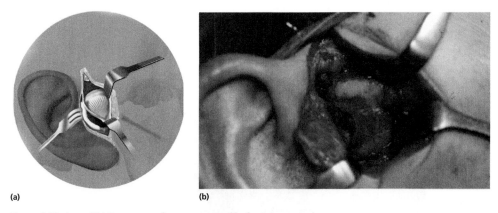

Figure 3.23 (a and b) Exposure of temporomandibular joint capsule.

Risdon submandibular approach was used mainly for open fracture reduction at the angle and body of the mandible. The approach to the joint is actually by way of a retro-mandibular incision, which allows superior retraction for placement of rigid fixation plates or screws for rib grafts or alloplastic implants. The incision is made on a curvilinear line approximately 5 cm long and 2 cm distal to the most inferior

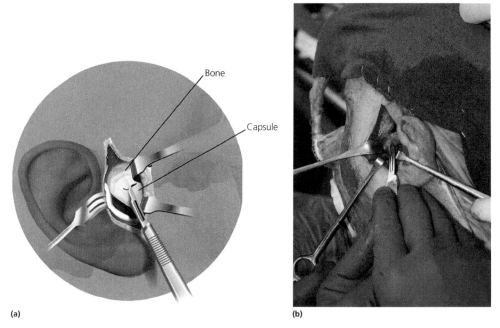

(a) (b)

Figure 3.24 (a and b) Entry into superior joint space. Blade is angled at 45° to avoid iatrogenic damage to the disk or condylar head.

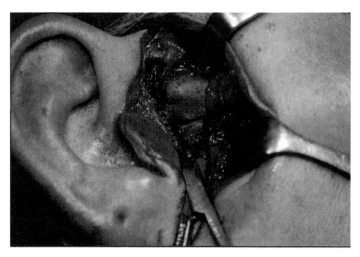

Figure 3.25 Curved hemostat used to open joint capsule and lyse joint adhesions.

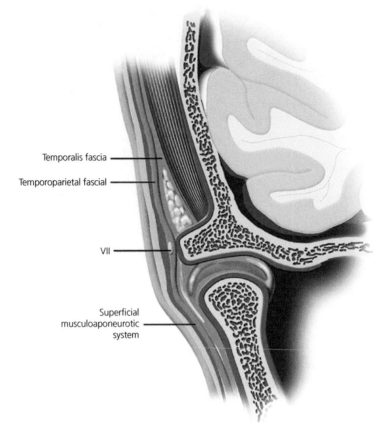

Figure 3.26 Coronal diagram of the fascial layers and facial nerve at the level of the temporoparietal fascial.

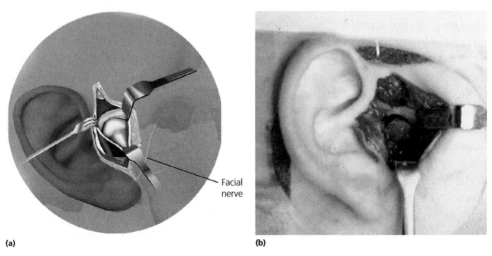

(a)   (b)

Figure 3.27 (a and b) Complete exposure of the temporomandibular joint. Note the careful positioning of the retractor on the zygomatic arch allowing protection of the retracted facial nerve.

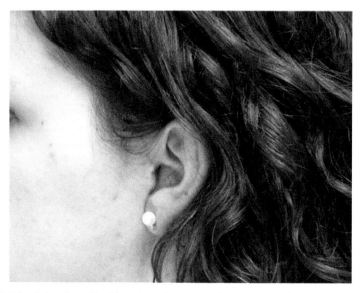

Figure 3.28 Well-healed endaural incision. Note the temporal extension within the hair line as well as the position of the tragal incision.

point of the mandibular angle, where its midpoint is situated. The incision is marked by placing a gloved finger from the lobule of the ear to the angle of the mandible. A marking pen is then used to identify the incision one-finger breadth below the angle of the mandible ensuring avoidance of the marginal mandibular nerve. The marginal mandibular branch of the facial nerve, posterior to the facial artery, passed above the inferior border of the mandible in 81% of dissections (Dingman and Grabb, 1962). It ran superficial to the facial vein in all the cadavers studied. It can, however, run as much as 3 cm below the inferior border of the mandible, deep to the platysma muscle. The dissection is carried down through skin, subcutaneous tissue, and platysma. A nerve stimulator is used to identify the mandibular branch, and it is retracted superiorly. Injury to the marginal mandibular nerve results in temporary or permanent denervation of the depressor anguli oris muscle. The patient is unable to depress the lower lip and show the mandibular anterior teeth. On the side of the injury, the affected side of the lip may appear to be pulled over the incisal edges of the teeth, as the normal side shows an exaggerated infero-lateral pull. The retromandibular vein (posterior facial vein) lies just behind the posterior border of the ramus lateral to the external carotid. Blunt dissection is used to define a plane between the sternocleidomastoid muscle and the capsule of the submandibular gland. Blunt finger dissection and retraction should be used to retract the anterior border of the

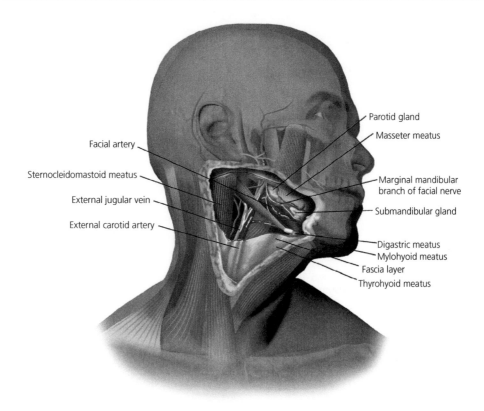

Parotid gland

Masseter meatus

Facial artery

Sternocleidomastoid meatus

Marginal mandibular branch of facial nerve

External jugular vein

Submandibular gland

External carotid artery

Digastric meatus
Mylohyoid meatus
Fascia layer
Thyrohyoid meatus

Figure 3.29 Critical anatomic structures encountered during the retromandibular approach to the mandible. Note the position of the facial nerve, and facial artery and vein to the angle of the mandible. The posterior belly of the digastric is deep to the mandible and runs at a 45° angle to the inferior border.

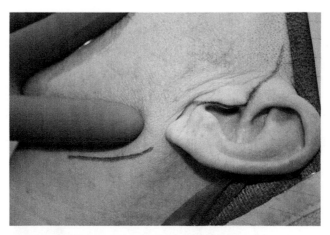

Figure 3.30 Marking of the modified retromandibular incision. Note superior extension on the incision in relation to the lobule of the ear.

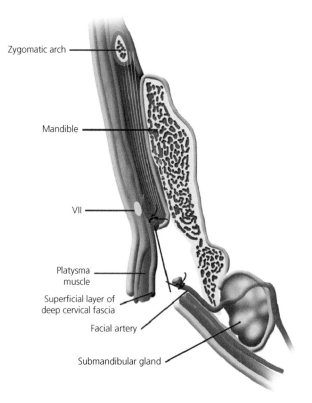

Zygomatic arch

Mandible

VII

Platysma muscle

Superficial layer of deep cervical fascia

Facial artery

Submandibular gland

Figure 3.31 Diagram demonstrating the relationship of the facial nerve and the artery to the mandible. The facial artery and vein often must be ligated to aid in exposure of the mandible.

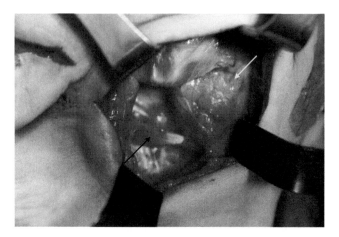

Figure 3.32 Retromandibular approach to the mandible. Note submandibular gland (yellow arrow) and posterior belly of the digastric (black arrow).

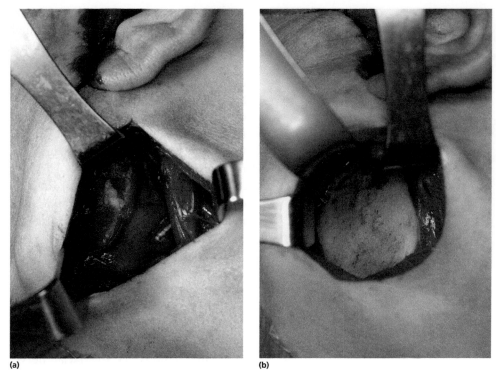

(a) (b)

Figure 3.33 (a) Retromandibular approach to the mandible with masseter exposed. (b) Exposure of mandible following dissection of the masseter. An incision is placed along the pterygomasseteric raphe and great care is taken to dissect the muscle from the mandible in a subperiosteal plane.

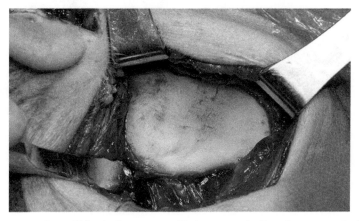

Figure 3.34 Exposure of mandible via the retromandibular approach. Note the communication between the endaural and retromandibular incisions.

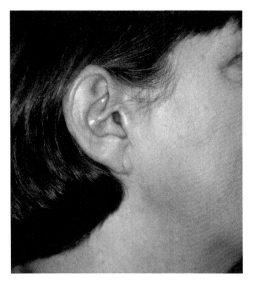

Figure 3.35 Well-healed endaural and retromandibular incisions following total joint replacement of the temporomandibular joint.

sternocleidomastoid posteriorly and the capsule of the submandibular gland anteriorly to visualize the aponeurosis of the masseter and the medial pterygoid along the inferior border of the ramus. A #15 blade is then used to make an incision through the aponeurosis. It is important to avoid incising through the body of the masseter muscle itself to prevent unnecessary hemorrhage. The masseter muscle can then be stripped off the lateral surface of the mandible, and with long right-angle retractors, the surgeon can visualize superiorly as far as the condylar neck and coronoid notch from this posterior-mandibular approach. This now allows communication between the two incisions in a safe subperiosteal plane. Care is taken to minimize trauma between the small cuffs of tissue between the two incisions, as the facial nerve travels in this plane.

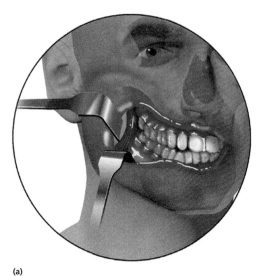

(a)

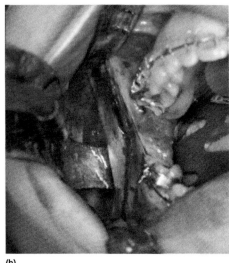

(b)

Figure 3.36 Diagram (a) and image (b) showing an intraoral approach to the temporomandibular joint.

Intraoral

An intraoral approach to the temporo-mandibular joint is achieved by making an incision along the external oblique ridge. A subperiosteal dissection proceeds medially and laterally along the mandibular ramus. A coronoid stripper may be used to remove the temporalis attachment from the coronoid to improve access. The coronoid process and condylar neck can be reached through this incision. Advantages of this approach include decreased facial and auriculotemporal nerve injury and improved scar placement. Limitations include limited access to the structures superior to the condylar neck. This approach can be useful in cases of fracture repair and may be considered for condylectomy.

Prep and positioning

Utilization of aseptic technique is crucial to minimize postoperative infection. A preoperative antibiotic should be given approximately 1 h before incision to ensure adequate tissue levels at the time of incision. Hair should be removed from the proposed incision site, typically to the level of the superior portion of the helix. Tape is then used to pull the remaining hair back and prevent its entry during the operation. A head wrap is applied and the skin is prepped. A urologic drape is then adapted and used as a sterile barrier to manipulate the mandible during the operation. The face and neck is then prepped. Once this is complete, the ear canal is irrigated with antibiotic solution; alternatively, a cotton pellet impregnated

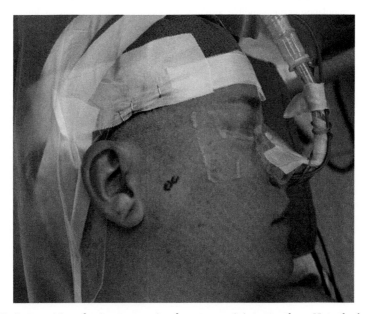

Figure 3.37 Patient positioned prior to prepping for an open joint procedure. Note the hair is removed to the level of the helix and 2-in. tape is used to prevent the remaining hair from entering the field.

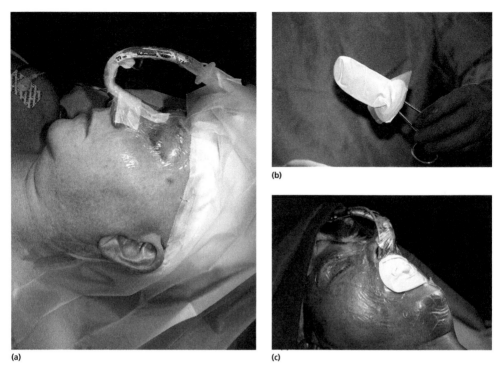

(a)

(b)

(c)

Figure 3.38 (a) Patient draped prior to prepping. (b) Modified urologic dressing. (c) Urologic dressings allowing sterile manipulation of the mandible, also note Tegaderm covering the nares to limit contamination.

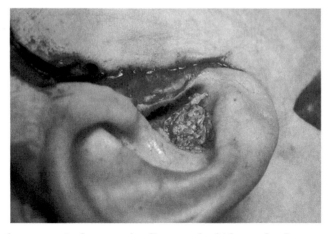

Figure 3.39 Note the cerumen in the external auditory canal, which can often be a source of contamination. A 60 cc syringe with normal saline and Webster cannula are used to irrigate the external auditory canal with antibiotic-impregnated saline. This allows the removal of debris from the ear.

with mineral oil can be placed within the external auditory canal.

References

Al-Kayat A, Bramley P. (1980) A modified pre-auricular approach to the temporomandibular joint and malar arch. *Br J Oral Surg*, 17:91.

Dingman RO, Grabb WC. (1962) Surgical anatomy of the mandibular ramus of the facial nerve, based on the dissection of 100 facial halves. *Plast Reconstr Sur*, 29:266.

Walters PJ, Geist ET. (1983) Correction of TMJ internal derangements by postauricular approach. *J Oral Maxillofac Surg*, 41:616.

Selected reading

Dolwick MF, Kretzschmar DP. (1982) Morbidity associated with preauricular and perimeatal approaches to the TMJ. *J Oral Maxillofac Surg*, 40:699.

Fujimura K. *et al.* (2006) Anatomical study of the complications of intraoral vertico-sagittal ramus osteotomy. *J Oral Maxillofac Surg*, 64:384.

Gordon SD. (1958) Surgery of the temporomandibular joint. *Am J Surg*, 95:263.

Hall MB. *et al.* (1985) Facial nerve injury during surgery of the temporomandibular joint: a comparison of dissection techniques. *J Oral Maxillofac Surg*, 43:20.

Ko EC. *et al.* (2009) Intraoral approach for arthroplasty for correction of TMJ ankylosis. *Int J Oral Maxillofac Surg*, 38:1256.

Talebzadeh N. *et al.* (1999) Anatomy of the structures medial to the temporomandibular joint. *Oral Surg Oral Med Oral Pathol Oral Radiol Endod*, 88:674.

CHAPTER 4
Surgery for internal derangements

Surgery for internal derangement is reserved for patients for whom nonsurgical conservative methods and arthroscopic techniques fail to control pain and increase functional range of motion. Because the temporomandibular joint (TMJ) is a ginglymoarthrodial joint with unique biomechanical demands, the mechanics of the disk-condyle complex may be extremely difficult to replicate with any surgical technique. Meniscal salvage procedures are usually confined to patients in Wilkes stages II and III but can occasionally be effective in stage IV as well. In stage V disease, the success rate of meniscal repair is clearly lower than in the earlier stages.

Open joint surgery ranges from meniscal repositioning to meniscectomy with or without replacement. Currently acceptable open joint procedures include the following: (i) meniscoplasty with or without arthroplasty, (ii) meniscectomy, (iii) meniscectomy with temporary silicone implant, (iv) meniscectomy with autogenous or allogeneic graft, (v) meniscectomy with condyloplasty or eminoplasty, (vi) repair of perforated posterior attachment with meniscal recontouring and repositioning, and (vii) modified mandibular condylotomy.

The main goal of all these procedures is to decrease pain and increase the range of motion. A reasonable goal is an interincisal opening of 35 mm with lateral excursions of 4–6 mm. Desirable functional outcomes would enable the patient to masticate a normal or nearly normal diet with a stable occlusion. In addition, open arthroplastic procedures can be expected to significantly reduce functionally induced pain.

As previously discussed, the joint is exposed through an endaural or preauricular incision. The surgeon may find it helpful to palpate the lateral pole of the condyle continually while the other hand uses a sterile urology drape as an intraoral manipulator. This allows the surgeon to constantly move the mandible to ascertain the exact position of the lateral pole and the palpable capsular depression between the glenoid fossa and the lateral pole. Once the capsule itself is isolated, a small amount of local anesthetic (1 ml) can be used to insufflate the joint space. The #15 blade is then used to make a small opening through the lateral capsule into the superior joint space. The blade is angled superiorly at approximately 45° to prevent any iatrogenic damage to the disk as it courses over the lateral pole to attach

Atlas of Temporomandibular Joint Surgery, Second Edition. Edited by Peter D. Quinn and Eric J. Granquist.
© 2015 John Wiley & Sons, Inc. Published 2015 by John Wiley & Sons, Inc.
Companion Website: www.wiley.com/go/quinn/atlasTMJsurgery

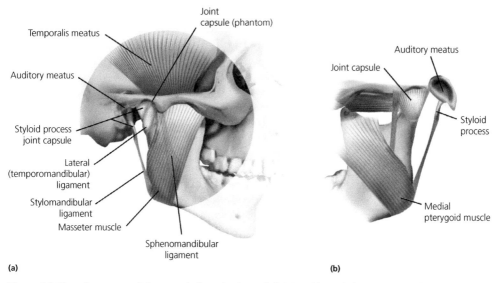

Figure 4.1 Note the extent of the capsule from both medial (a) and lateral (b) views. On the lateral view, the temporomandibular ligament extends across the inferior insertion of the capsule.

Table 4.1 Wilkes classification for internal derangement of the TMJ.

Stage	Characteristics	Imaging
I. Early	Painless clicking	Slight forward disk
	No restricted motion	Normal osseous contours
II. Early/intermediate	Occasional painful clicking	Slight forward disk
	Intermittent locking	Early disk deformity
	Headaches	Normal osseous contours
III. Intermediate	Frequent pain	Anterior disk displacement
	Joint tenderness	Moderate to marked disk thickening
	Headaches, locking	Normal osseous contours
	Restricted motion	
	Painful chewing	
IV. Intermediate/late	Chronic pain, headache	Anterior disk displacement
	Restricted motion	Marked disk thickening
		Abnormal bone contours
V. Late	Variable pain, joint	Anterior disk displacement with disk
	crepitus	perforation and gross deformity
		Degenerative osseous changes

to the capsule. An assistant may depress the posterior molars inferiorly to increase the joint space during this maneuver. The small hemostat may be used to widen the opening into the superior joint space. The egress of synovial fluid should confirm immediately that the surgeon is in the superior joint space.

The #15 blade is again used to open up the incision from a posterior and

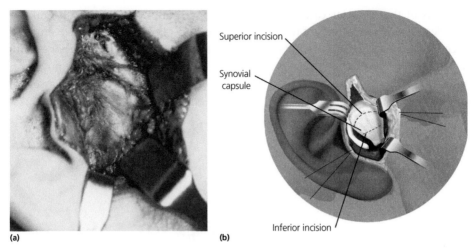

Figure 4.2 (a) Capsule of the right temporomandibular joint. The surgeon can easily palpate the lateral pole of the condyle and superior joint space by feeling for the depression between the glenoid fossa and the condyle. (b) Diagram of the right temporomandibular joint capsule. Note the position of the superior incision (to enter the superior joint space) and inferior incision (to enter the inferior joint space).

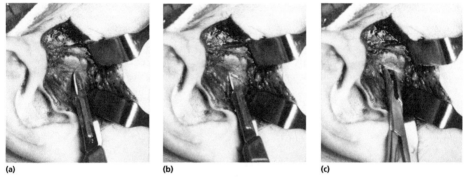

Figure 4.3 Series of photos showing incision of the joint capsule and entry into the superior joint space. Note that #15 blade is at angle 45° to avoid injuring the disk. Once the incision is made into the joint capsule, the capsule can further be dissected open with the aid of a curved hemostat.

an anterior point to visualize the entire superior surface of the disk and the anterior and posterior recesses of the joint space. A small freer elevator can be used to sweep gently across the top of the disk to break any adhesions at this point. In joints on which no previous surgery has been performed, this procedure is relatively easy. In joints that have undergone multiple operations, however, this can be a complicated dissection, especially with the presence of fibrous ankylosis.

After obtaining adequate visualization of the joint space, the surgeon must immediately evaluate the disk position before the mechanics of the surgery falsely alter it. This is also the opportunity to determine whether the disk or the posterior attachment is perforated. The surrounding tissues can be examined for synovitis, fibrillations of the articular cartilage, and any evidence of osteoarthrosis of the bony surfaces. Removal of the lateral third of the articular eminence with a small osteotome is sometimes helpful to improve visualization within the anterior joint space. This maneuver also increases the lateral joint space and allows for freer movement of the disk. At this point, adhesions in the superior joint space can be removed and the joint can be manipulated to assess the mechanics of the condyle-disk complex.

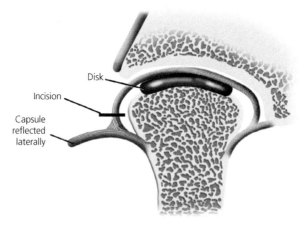

Figure 4.4 Incision into inferior joint space is made at the neck of the condyle, just above the inferior attachment of the lateral ligament. Once the incision is made, a nasal freer can be used to disk free the disk. Care should be taken to avoid damaging the fibrocartilage covering the condyle.

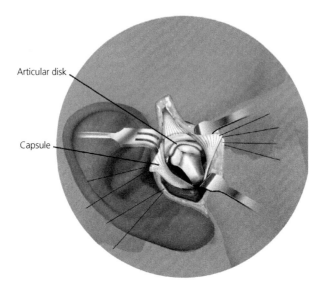

Figure 4.5 Incision of both superior and inferior joint spaces to isolate the disk for either repair or meniscectomy.

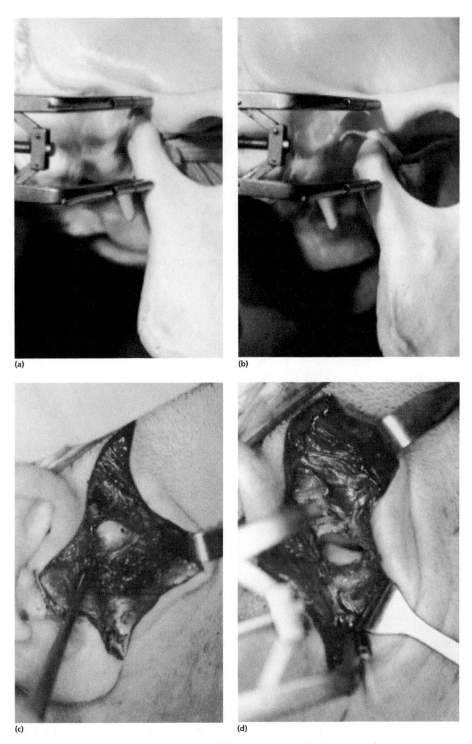

Figure 4.6 (a–c) In order to improve exposure of the temporomandibular joint and superior joint space, a Wilkes retractor can be utilized. The Wilkes retractor is secured into the zygomatic arch superiorly and condylar neck inferiorly with Kirschner wires (a and b). This then allows for retraction of the condyle from the glenoid fossa improving access (c and d).

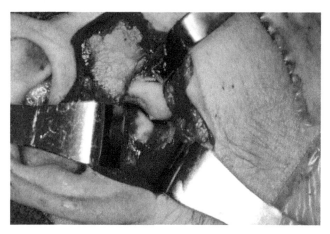

Figure 4.7 Open view of the superior joint space showing normal dimensions of the anterior recess with the anterior attachment of the capsule intact along the anterior aspect of the articular eminence.

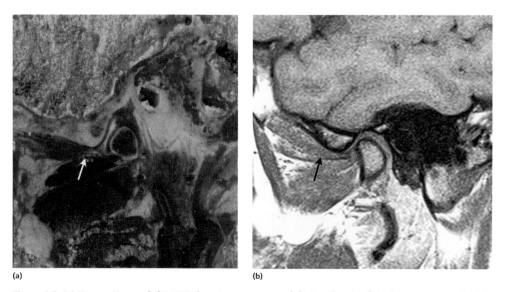

(a)   (b)

Figure 4.8 (a) Cryosection and (b) MRI showing separate and distinct heads of the lateral pterygoid with fat plane separation.

The surgeon should observe closely for folding of the meniscus during opening and closing or obstructions to normal disk movement from the articular eminence. The surgeon must assess the disk in its total medial-lateral dimension and ensure that no adhesions are present on the medial surface that would make it difficult to position the disk posteriorly and laterally. In rare cases, this exposure into the superior joint space may be all that is necessary if the main problem was adhesion of the disk to the articular eminence or isolated adhesions in the superior joint

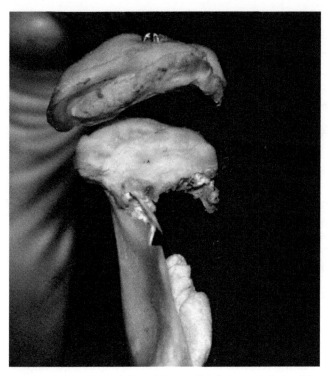

Figure 4.9 Cadaver specimen showing condyle and dissected disk. Note medial and lateral extension of the disk. During meniscal procedures the surgeon should appreciate this dimension so that adequate dissection is performed deep enough on the medial surface to free any potential adhesions so that the surgeon can remove the entire disk.

space. If the condyle and disk function properly after these maneuvers, the joint space can be irrigated and the incision can be closed.

Some surgeons prefer to use a temporary silicone implant to prevent adhesions of the disk to the glenoid fossa and articular eminence. In most cases, the inferior joint space must also be explored. Palpation of the neck of the condyle just above the insertion of the capsule is critical. The #15 blade is again used to make a small incision through the capsule inferior to the disk itself. A small periosteal elevator is used to widen this incision and then the freer elevator is used to free the lateral meniscal attachment. The same elevator is then used to sweep over the top of the condyle to free the disk from an inferior approach. Prevention of any direct trauma to the fibrocartilage on the condylar head is always important during these maneuvers. The approach to the inferior joint space can be widened anteriorly and posteriorly with a small Iris or Metzenbaum scissors. The condyle is now examined from the inferior approach for the presence of degeneration and osteophytes. Although condyloplasty is rarely employed because of the inability of the condylar bone

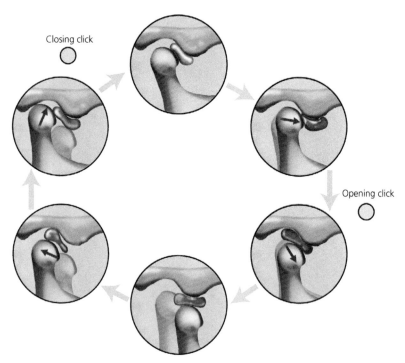

Figure 4.10 Representation of reciprocal clicking, secondary to anterior displacement with reduction.

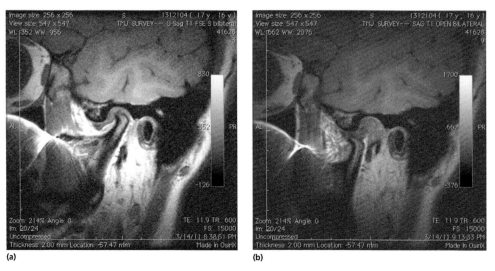

Figure 4.11 (a) T1 MRI in the closed position showing anteriorly displaced disk. Note thickening of the retrodiscal tissue and "bird beaking" of the condyle. (b) T1 MRI in the open position. Note reduction of the disk on opening.

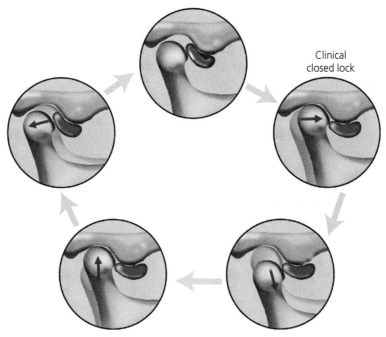

Clinical
closed lock

Figure 4.12 Diagram showing an anteriorly displaced disk without reduction. Note loss of translation of the condyle and absence of opening or closing click.

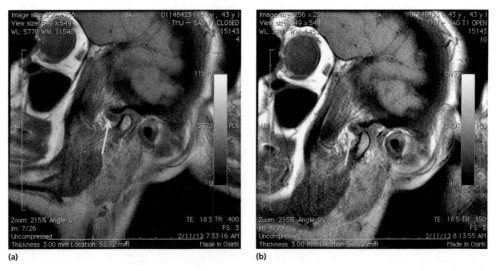

(a)   (b)

Figure 4.13 T1 MRI closed position (a) and open position (b). Note anteriorly displaced disk with loss of biconcave "bow-tie" shape (arrow) and minimal translation of condylar head in the open MRI (b).

to repair itself after surgical trauma, the contouring of gross deformities is sometimes necessary. This can be done with a diamond bur under copious irrigation. A small freer elevator can also be used to explore the inferior surface of the disk to diagnose any perforations that may not have been visible from the superior joint space. A decision must be made at this point regarding the type of procedure that will be performed on the disk. The surgical options are as follows: (i) disk plication—surgical repositioning of the disk by suturing it to retrodiscal and lateral capsular tissues, (ii) diskopexy— a disk "tie-down" that anchors the disk to a condylar or fossa purchase point, (iii) lysis of adhesions in both superior and inferior joint spaces without any disk repositioning (the last procedure can be performed in conjunction with eminoplasty), and (iv) meniscectomy (discectomy) with or without replacement. A Wilkes retractor may be used to aid in visualization and access to the disc by placing Kirschner wires in the zygomatic arch and the neck of the condyle. The retractor can then fit over the cut ends of the Kirschner wires and retract the condyle inferiorly and anteriorly.

In the disk repositioning procedures, the surgeon must sometimes release the disk anteriorly by using a #15 blade or electrocautery to incise the anterior attachment in the area of the anterior capsular wall. Theoretically, this technique lessens the anterior and medial pull of the lateral pterygoid muscle.

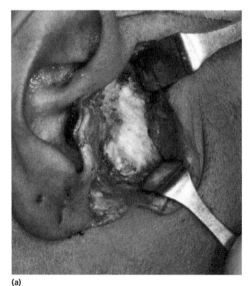
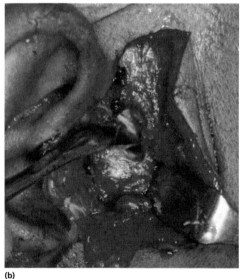

(a)　　　　　　　　　　　　(b)

Figure 4.14 (a) Endaural approach to temporomandibular joint showing intact capsule of temporomandibular joint. (b) Exposure into superior joint space showing marked adhesions from superior surface of the articular disk to the glenoid fossa.

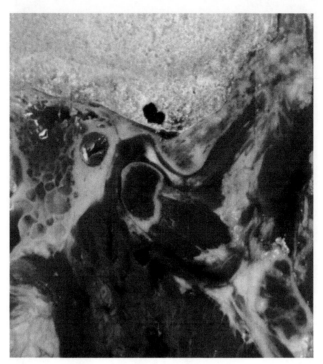

Figure 4.15 Cyrosection showing normal physiologic position of meniscus with relationship to anterior–superior slope of the condyle and articular eminence. Note that the junction of the posterior attachment and the posterior band of the disk is approximately at the 12 o'clock position on the condylar head. Also note the normal dimensions of the functioning disk, which are 3 mm anterior band, 1 mm intermediate zone, and 2 mm posterior band.

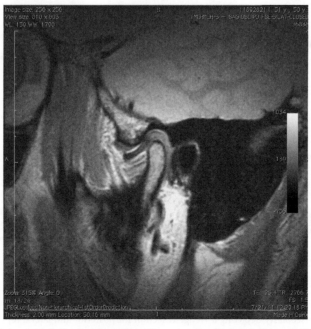

Figure 4.16 MRI of the condyle in closed position. Note anterior displaced disk and slight thickening of the retrodiscal tissue.

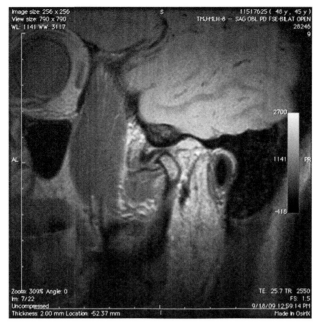

Figure 4.17 MRI of the condyle in the open position. Note the disk is anteriorly displaced and does not reduce. Also note the loss of the normal 3-1-2 biconcave disk shape and degeneration of the condylar head.

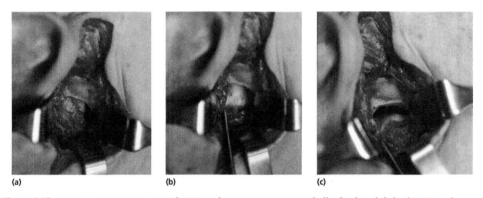

(a) (b) (c)

Figure 4.18 (a) Superior joint space, right joint, showing anterior-medially displaced disk. (b) Tissue forceps pulling displaced disk in exaggerated lateral position. (c) Tissue forceps holding repositioned meniscus in lateral-posterior position, which allows unrestricted motion of condyle without clicking or locking.

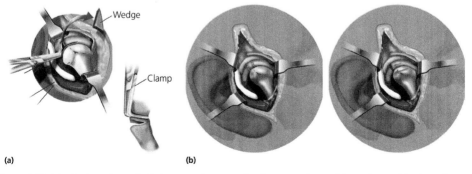

(a) (b)

Figure 4.19 (a) Meniscoplasty depicting a wedge resection for posterior and lateral repositioning of an anterior-medially displaced meniscus. The dimension of the wedge can be altered to control the vector of pull and final position of the disk. Note the use of a right-angle tissue clamp, which can aid in the control of bleeding. (b) Prior to resection of posterior attachment (outlined). Note the edges of the resection must be in vascular tissue to ensure healing.

Disk plication

Disk plication can be either a complete or a partial procedure. In the complete disk plication, a full wedge of retrodiscal tissues is removed and the disk is repositioned by suturing the remaining retrodiscal tissue directly to the posterior ligament.

In a partial plication, a small, pie-shaped wedge of tissue is removed to facilitate repositioning in a simultaneous posterior and lateral plane. Separation of the condyle from the fossa allows better visibility and increased working space for surgical instruments.

In the plication procedure, specially modified right-angle vascular clamps are used to clamp the anterior and posterior attachments at the level of the wedge resection. This provides both hemostasis

and control of the soft tissue edges. The repair is performed with multiple resorbable 4-0 sutures on a small curved needle. It is helpful to pass all the sutures first rather than tying them down sequentially, which can limit subsequent suture placement. The goal is to replicate as closely as possible the normal position of the disk.

In most cases, this means that the junction of the posterior attachment and posterior band of the disk are at approximately the 12 o'clock position with reference to the condylar curve. After the repair, many surgeons find it helpful to simulate a range of motion with the condyle to ensure the absence of mechanical obstruction, catching, or locking.

At this point, the surgeon should determine whether an anterior release should be performed with electrocautery, laser, or

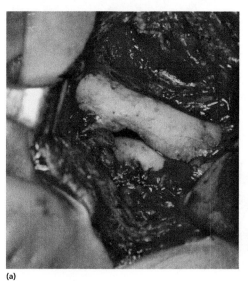 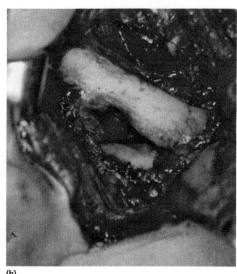

(a)   (b)

Figure 4.20 (a) Note repositioned meniscus in closed position. Suture line is visible along lateral capsular attachment. It is preferable to keep the suture knots away from any area that would possibly be in contact during joint loading. (b) Note the condyle is maneuvered after the disk repair is complete to ensure smooth condyle-disk function during the expected range of motion. No excessive pull should occur on the suture line at the terminal opening point.

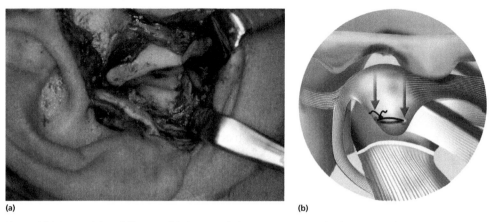

(a)   (b)

Figure 4.21 Image (a) and diagram (b) showing disk repositioning to the lateral attachment.

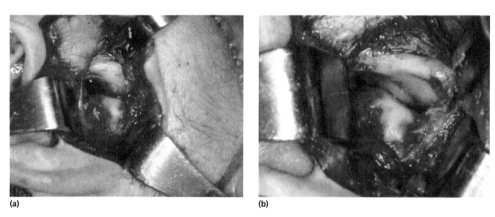

(a)   (b)

Figure 4.22 (a) Case in which an eminoplasty was used as an isolated procedure for the treatment of chronic open lock. (b) Note the increased joint space with condyle in closed position.

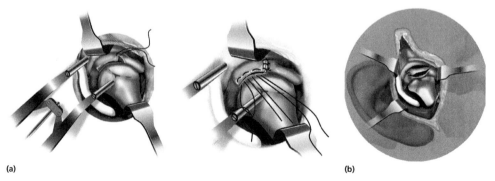

(a)   (b)

Figure 4.23 Meniscoplasty depicting a wedge resection for posterior and lateral repositioning of an anterior-medially displaced disk (a). The dimensions of the wedge can be altered to control the vector of movement of the disk. Once the disk is repositioned posteriorly-laterally (lower diagram), the lateral repair can proceed (b). A curved scissors or electrocautery is used to release the anterior attachment near the anterior capsular wall for a tension-free repositioning of the disk. Simple interrupted or horizontal mattress 4-0 sutures are used.

small surgical scissors. When the condyle is secured in a satisfactory position, the surgeon can decide whether an eminoplasty should be performed to increase the superior joint space if mechanical obstruction is still present. In the partial-thickness technique, a complete resection of the posterior attachment is usually unnecessary, but excess lateral capsular tissue can be excised with scissors, and a small wedge of tissue is removed to help position the disk in a more lateral-posterior position.

Diskopexey

Condylar diskopexey is a procedure in which the displaced disk is freed by the surgeon entering both joint spaces and lysing adhesions first. At this point, a small hole is placed through the lateral pole of the condyle from posterior to anterior. A nonresorbable 2-0 or 3-0 suture is placed through the hole and through the disk at the junction of the anterior and intermediate bands. Four to five additional 4-0 nonresorbable sutures are then placed from the lateral surface of the disk to the lateral capsular attachment on the condyle. If deformity of the disk precludes repositioning it into a more normal position, recontouring the thickened disk with a scalpel is sometimes necessary. This recontouring can also be performed with the operating microscope.

Some surgeons favor the use of a temporal diskopexey for stage III and stage IV internal derangements when the disk is too deformed to function in a condyle-disk unit. In this case, the disk is secured to the roof of the glenoid fossa by placing two bur holes in the posterolateral lip of the fossa. The patient should be assessed preoperatively with MRI studies and intraoperatively to judge the repairability of the disk. Although attempts to salvage late-stage meniscal displacements are losing favor, the success of the disk repair depends on the degree of deformity and the extent of degenerative changes at the time of the arthroplasty. In some cases of disk deformity, a simultaneous eminoplasty to increase the superior joint space may be appropriate. After the plication is completed, the mandible is manipulated to assess the area on the eminence where the disk impinges. The condyle is then separated from the fossa, and a large diamond bur is used to contour the eminence to allow unobstructed passage of the condyle-disk complex. Care is taken to avoid removing the fibrocartilage in the fossa itself during this maneuver. Some surgeons recommend use of a temporary silicone implant after this procedure to prevent the disk from adhering to the surface of the recontoured articular eminence.

Another technique for securing the disk in a more physiologic position is the use of the Mitek anchor. This bone-anchoring system allows a metal insert to be placed inside the condylar head with a suture attached to it. This system is commonly used for knee surgery. In this technique, the Mitek drill is used to create a hole in the posterior-lateral surface of the condylar neck. The Mitek bone-cleat introducer is inserted and pushed into the bone, where two small coils unlock and attach the cleat to the inner surface of the cortical bone. The nonresorbable woven suture is then passed with a fine needle through the free edge of the disk, and the disk is tied down to the condylar neck.

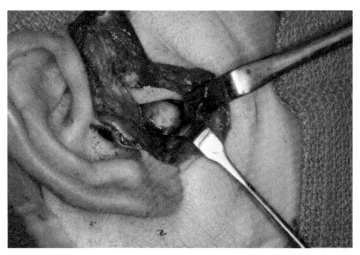

Figure 4.24 Meniscal repositioning posteriorly-laterally after anterior release (with eminoplasty).

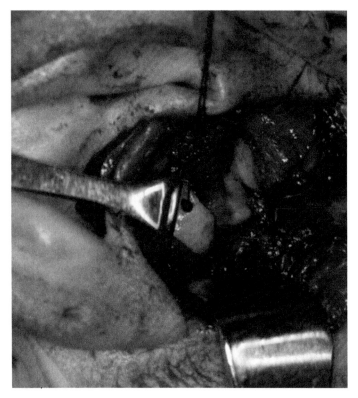

Figure 4.25 Nonresorbable suture used to secure a displaced disk to a hole in the lateral pole of the condyle (anchor procedure preferable).

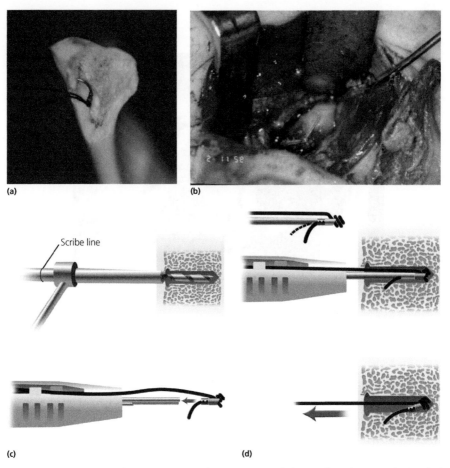

Figure 4.26 (a) Sectioned condylar specimen to show insertion of the Mitek anchor into the head of the condyle from a posterior–lateral approach. (b) Repositioned disk held in position by Mitek anchor. (c, d) Diagram of insertion of Mitek anchor into condylar head for meniscal repositioning procedure.

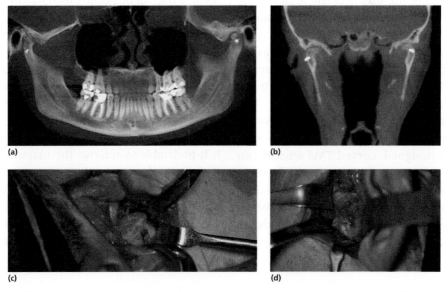

Figure 4.27 Panorex (a) and coronal CT (b) showing Mitek anchoring system in place. (c and d) Intraoperative views of the same patient showing the Mitek anchors in place prior to total alloplastic joint replacement.

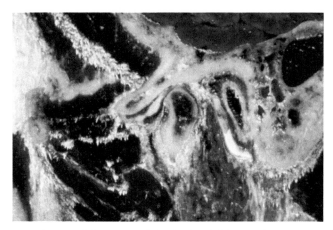

Figure 4.28 Cryosection showing deformation of the displaced disk as well as sclerosis of the anterior slope of the condylar head.

Meniscectomy (discectomy)

Meniscectomy can be performed when the disk is irreparable. Many surgeons favor meniscectomy for internal derangement as the primary surgical treatment following the failure of medical and arthroscopic interventions, or when perforations are noted on arthroscopic exam. Meniscectomy is the removal of the central avascular portion of the disk and the area of perforation through the posterior ligament, where the tissues may be irreparably damaged. Most surgeons leave a small amount of anterior and posterior attachment to prevent excessive hemorrhage with resultant fibrosis. The most difficult portion of the disk to remove is its medial extension. A specially designed, curved TMJ scissors can be used to cut the anterior and posterior attachments. The bleeding can then be controlled with packs of thrombin-soaked sponges and a local anesthesia containing epinephrine.

The final step is accomplished by using a Wilkes retractor to retract the condyle in an anterior-inferior direction. This allows maximal access to the medial recess. Either the curved TMJ scissors or a # 15 blade is used to separate the disk from its medial attachment. The surgeon must be careful not to cut through the medial capsular wall and damage the middle meningeal artery.

Once the disk is removed, the joint space can again be packed with thrombin-soaked sponges until hemostasis is obtained. One of the most common reasons for meniscectomy is perforation of the disk itself. As mentioned previously, a small freer elevator can be used to explore the disk from the inferior joint space, and check for perforations that may not be visible on initial entry into the joint space. It is preferable to remove the majority of the meniscal tissue and trim any loose, irregular edges at the margins of the meniscectomy to prevent potential adhesions and fibrosis. Controversy exists in the literature about the type of reconstructive

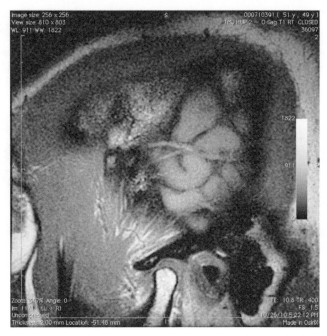

Figure 4.29 MRI showing thinning of the disk and possible perforation.

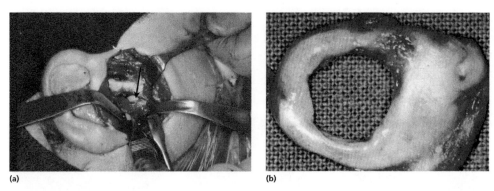

(a) (b)

Figure 4.30 (a) Large perforation with visualization of the condylar head (arrow). (b) Large perforation through postero-central portion of the meniscus.

procedure that should be performed after meniscectomy. Some researchers advocate meniscectomy alone without replacement, and some long-term follow-up studies of these procedures show that patients can experience marked pain relief with an adequate range of motion.

Universally, adaptive changes are apparent, even in successful meniscectomies, which appear radiographically as flattening of the anterior–superior slope of the condyle with sclerosis and some beaking of the anterior lip of the condyle. Crepitus is also a common finding after meniscectomy

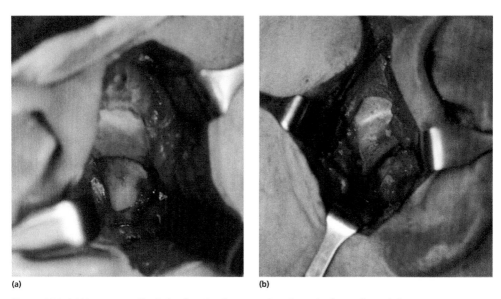

(a)   (b)

Figure 4.31 (a) Temporary silastic implant in place covering the articular surface of the temporomandibular joint. (b) Temporary silastic in place, note superior extension placed under the temporalis fascia.

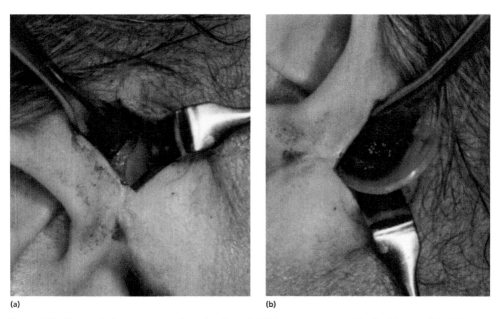

(a)   (b)

Figure 4.32 Removal of a temporary silastic implant. (a) This can be accomplished with a small "nick" incision along the superior aspect of the previous incision. The implant should be carefully removed while an assistant is pulling the mandible inferiorly to minimize pressure on the implant and prevent tearing (b). The implant should be carefully inspected following removal to ensure it was removed in its entirety.

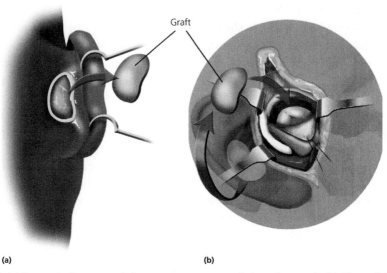

Figure 4.33 (a) Postauricular approach for an autogenous conchal cartilage graft. (b) The graft is then secured and contoured into the surface of the glenoid fossa.

without replacement. Several MRI studies have shown the development of a "pseudo" disk or scar tissue formation between the condyle and glenoid fossa.

A technique described by Wilkes is the use of the temporary silicone "pull-out" implant. The medical-grade silicone sheeting is contoured into an ovoid intra-articular interpositional implant with a temporal extension that can be placed under the superficial or deep temporalis fascia. The silicone forms a heavy fibrous capsule and, when used in this short-term fashion, does not appear to cause any foreign-body type of reactions. When silicone was used as a permanent implant in the joint, documented reactions included silicone synovitis and giant cell-mediated foreign-body reactions that were caused by the particulation of the material during excessive wear. Even in that event the reactions were not as aggressive as those seen with the polytetrafluoroethylene (PTFE) implants.

The temporary silicone implants prevent adhesions between the condyle and the glenoid fossa and promote the formation of a fibrous tissue lining, which can separate the bony articular surfaces of the joint. Once the temporary silicone implant is in place, the surgeon should move the mandible to ensure that all the articular surfaces are covered by the implant and that motion does not displace the implant from the glenoid fossa. The surgeon must remove the implant, and this can be performed as an office procedure with intravenous sedation and local anesthesia. The implant is generally removed approximately 6–12 weeks after surgery, but removal can be delayed for several months beyond this point if the patient's condition warrants that decision. It is reasonable to remove the implant when the interincisal opening is approximately 35 mm and the patient's pain level has decreased to a level at which narcotic medications are unnecessary. A small incision, which is 1–1.5 cm, is sufficient to remove the silicone implant. Care should be taken to free the tissue encapsulating the silastic sheet, as well as distract the condyle inferiorly prior to removal of the implant. This will minimize tearing. It is essential to inspect the implant for tears and irregularities to confirm its complete removal. Retained foreign bodies will necessitate exploration of the joint to ensure all materials have been removed. An alternative to placing any alloplastic material after meniscectomy is to inject the pateint's own platelet-rich plasma into the joint space to fill the "dead space" and accelerate healing.

Meniscectomy with replacement

Autogenous, allogeneic, and alloplastic materials have all been used to replace the disk after meniscectomy. Long-term studies of patients with meniscectomy without replacement indicate that some patients do very well without any tissue replacement. It is equally obvious that no viable alloplastic disk-implant material is available at this time. The well-documented severe pathologic responses to PTFE interpositional implants and, to a lesser degree, permanent silicone implants clearly negate this approach.

Of the autogenous tissues, the three most commonly used are dermis, auricular cartilage, and temporalis fascia and/or temporalis muscle. Allogeneic materials such as fascia, dura, and cartilage have been used, but autogenous materials have the advantage of obviating the possibility of antigenicity or infectious disease transmission.

Dermal graft

The dermal graft can be harvested "freehand" in the lateral thigh or abdomen. An elliptical incision is made to excise the full-thickness graft with both epidermis and dermis intact. The graft should measure approximately 3–4 cm by 3 cm, and a #15 blade is used to remove the epidermal layer. Because the graft tends to contract during harvesting and handling, the piece of tissue excised should be larger than the actual dimensions of the meniscal defect and be harvested in a "non-hair-bearing" area.

Another technique to harvest the dermal graft is to use a dermatone to create a full-thickness skin graft that is not detached at its base. The dermal graft is then harvested, and the skin graft is repositioned and sutured at the periphery. Some authors advocate using the #15 blade to make "quilting-type" cuts through the skin graft to prevent displacement by a subepithelial hematoma. Once the dermis is prepared, it is placed into the joint space and sutured to both remnants of the anterior and posterior attachment with 4-0 resorbable suture.

Auricular cartilage

Auricular cartilage has also been used as a disk replacement and can be harvested by a posterior approach that leaves a very acceptable scar. Designing the incision so that it will cover intact cartilage after the graft is removed is extremely important. An attempt is made to harvest cartilage with a curvilinear shape so that it will match the contour of the glenoid fossa. Usually the cartilage must be secured to several small holes drilled on the lateral-inferior lip of the glenoid fossa. In harvesting the graft, surgeons must be

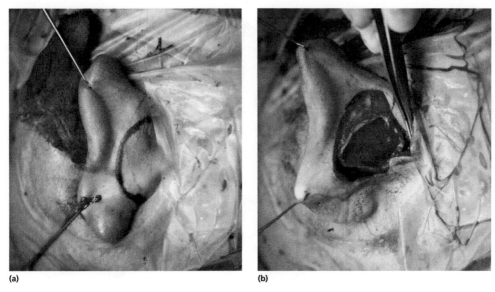

(a)   (b)

Figure 4.34 (a) Posterior approach to ear to harvest auricular cartilage. The incision is approximately 4 cm. (b) The incision is placed between the antihelix and the outer helix. The incision is positioned so that it will remain over intact cartilage after graft harvesting. The graft removed should be smaller in diameter than the distance between the incision and the mastoid crease. Hemostasis must be achieved to prevent an auricular hematoma postoperatively.

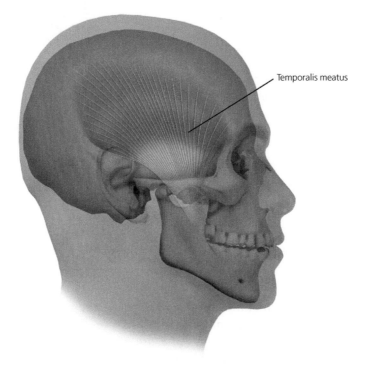

Temporalis meatus

Figure 4.35 Diagram of temporalis muscle. A myofascial or facial flap may be used as a graft to replace the temporomandibular disk and prevent ankylosis.

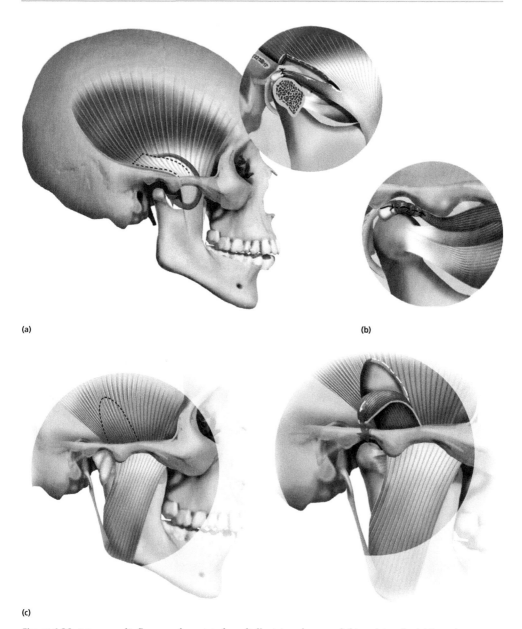

(a)

(b)

(c)

Figure 4.36 A temporalis flap may be rotated medially (a) and secured (b) or laterally (c) into the glenoid fossa.

careful not to violate the rim of the anti-helix during graft removal. They must also remember to dissect the perichondrium off the graft on the lateral surface and maintain the perichondrium on the medial surface. Some surgeons advocate the use of a temporary silicone implant for approximately 6 weeks to prevent

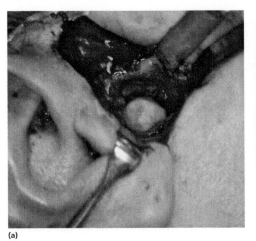 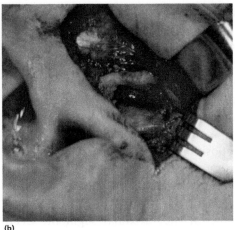

(a)   (b)

Figure 4.37 (a and b) Status post-meniscectomy with temporalis fascia graft in position. Graft is sutured anteriorly to the anterior aspect of the capsular ligament and the lateral pterygoid muscle and posteriorly to the posterior attachment.

adhesions between the condyle and the auricular graft. Use of a small rubber drain in the postauricular ear wound and a pressure dressing to prevent an auricular hematoma is of utmost importance.

Temporalis muscle and fascial grafts

Temporalis fascia was used as a free autogenous interpositional graft in the past but has largely been abandoned in favor of the temporalis myofascial flap because the fascia alone proved insufficient in mass to function adequately. The temporalis myofascial flap is harvested by extending the endaural incision into the temporal region approximately 2–3 cm. This interiorly based, full-thickness flap incorporating the muscle with superficial and deep fascia, is outlined and freed with a #15 blade or a cautery tip. To account for contraction, the distal width of the flap should be wider than the actual dimensions of the joint space to

be covered. In general, the length of the flap from the superior edge to the zygomatic arch is 5–6 cm and approximately 3 cm in width. The edges of the flap are then sewed together with multiple 4-0 chromic sutures. The flap is rotated laterally over the zygomatic arch and placed as a lining into the glenoid fossa so that the periosteum from the temporal bone is facing against the glenoid fossa. The flap is held in position with two nonresorbable sutures that are passed through holes drilled in the posterior edge of the fossa and the bone on the anterior slope of the eminence.

An alternative method for placing the temporalis flap is to raise the same inferiorly based temporalis myofascial flap, bring the free edge through the infratemporal space, and pass it from the articular eminence posteriorly into the joint space. Once it is passed under the articular eminence, it is sutured to the rim of the glenoid fossa in a similar fashion.

Modified condylotomy

Another method for treating internal derangements, which Hall and others have popularized, is the modified condylotomy. This procedure can he used for internal derangements instead of conventional intracapsular disk-repositioning techniques. In essence, an intraoral vertical subsigmoid osteotomy is performed. A large pineapple bur is used to contour the lingual cortical bone of the proximal segment. Even though there is incomplete stripping of the medial pterygoid muscle, inferior and anterior repositioning of the proximal segment occurs. This allows the condyle to reposition itself in a more normal relationship with the displaced disk. This condylar movement is secondary to a shortening of the lateral pterygoid muscle, and the condylar repositioning essentially reduces the impingement on the retrodiscal tissues. A short period of intermaxillary fixation is followed by functional training with interarch elastics.

Postoperative care

Postoperative care is clearly an important aspect of any intracapsular joint surgery. Aggressive and early mobilization of the joint is tantamount to success. In most patients, regardless of the type of surgical procedure, progressive mobilization, with active motion exercises, is adequate to achieve an interincisal opening of approximately 35 mm within 4–6 weeks of surgery. Handheld jaw-exercise devices are available to assist patients in achieving this goal. In patients who have had multiple operations or continued problems with adhesions or heterotopic bone formation, a continuous passive motion device, in conjunction with active physiotherapy, can be helpful. In general, mobilization without mastication-induced joint loading should be encouraged for the first few weeks after surgery. A soft diet is usually advocated in the first 4–6 weeks following surgery. Once an adequate, pain-free interincisal opening is achieved, the diet can be rapidly advanced.

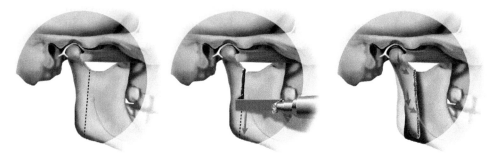

Figure 4.38 Intraoral vertical subsigmoid osteotomy. Note the improvement in the condyle-disk relationship after the anterior-inferior displacement of the proximal osteotomy segment.

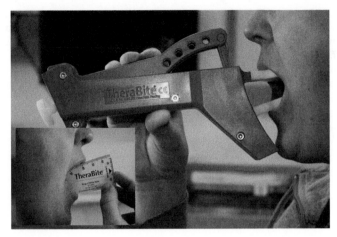

Figure 4.39 Patient demonstrating use of a TheraBite jaw exerciser. Patients are instructed to use a handheld jaw mobilization device three to four times daily for a period of 4–6 weeks. Patients can monitor their progress by measuring their maximal incisal opening (inset).

Suggested reading

Abramowicz S, Dolwick MF. (2010) 20-year follow-up of disc repositioning surgery for temporomandibular joint internal derangement. *J Oral Maxillofac Surg*, 68:239.

Annandale T. (1887) On displacement of the interarticular cartilage of the lower jaw and its treatment by operation. *Lancet*, 1:411.

Braun T. (1989) Temporomandibular joint surgery: surgical treatment of internal derangement. *Selected Readings Oral Maxillofac Surg*, 1:3.

Braun T. (1989/1990) Temporomandibular joint surgery, part 2. *Selected Readings Oral Maxillofac Surg*, 1:3; 1:4.

Costen JB. (1934) Syndrome of ear and sinus symptoms dependent upon disturbed function of the temporomandibular joint. *Ann Otol Rhinol Laryngol*, 43:1.

Dimitroulis G. (2011) A critical review of interpositional grafts following temporomandibular joint discectomy with an overview of the dermis-fat graft. *Int J Oral Maxillofac Surg*, 40:561.

Dolwick MF, Riggs RR. (1983) Diagnosis and treatment of internal derangements of the temporomandibular joint. *Dent Clin North Am*, 27:561

Eriksson L, Westesson P. (1985) Long-term evaluation of meniscectomy of the temporomandibular joint. *J Oral Maxillofac Surg*, 43:263.

Farrar WB, McCarty WL Jr. (1982) *A clinical outline for temporomandibular joint diagnosis and treatment*, ed 9, Normandie Publications, Montgomery, AL.

Feinberg SE. (1994/1985) Use of composite temporalis muscle flap for disc replacement. *Oral Maxillofac Surg Clin North Am*, 6:335; 78:569.

Hall HD, Link JL. (1989) Discectomy alone and with ear cartilage interpositional grafts in joint reconstruction. *Oral Maxillofac Clin North Am*, 1:329.

Hall HD. et al. (1993) Modified condylotomy for treatment of the painful temporomandibular joint with a reducing disc. *J Oral Maxillofac Surg*, 51:133.

Lanz W. (1909) Discitis mandibularis. *Zentralbl Chir*, 36:289.

Merrill RG. (1986) Histological perspectives and comparisons of TMJ surgery for internal disc derangements and arthropathy. *Cranio*, 4:75.

Miloro M, Henriksen B. (2010) Discectomy as the primary surgical option for internal derangement of the temporomandibular joint. *J Oral Maxillofac Surg*, 68:782.

Nickerson JW Jr. (1994) The role of condylotomy in the management of temporomandibular joint disorders. In *Controversies in oral and maxillofacial surgery* (Eds P Worthington and JR Evans). WB Saunders, Philadelphia.

Tucker MR. *et al.* (1990) Autogenous auricular cartilage implantation following discectomy in the temporomandibular joint. *J Oral Maxillofac Surg*, 48:38.

Werther JR. *et al.* (1995) Disk position before and after modified condylotomy in 80 symptomatic temporomandibular joints. *Oral Surg Oral Med Oral Path*, 79:668.

Wilkes CH. (1978) Structural and functional alterations of the temporomandibular joint. *Northwest Dent*, 57:287.

CHAPTER 5

Osseous surgery of the temporomandibular joint

Condyloplasty

Several authors have popularized the technique of condyloplasty, or condylar shave. Arthroplasty is the reshaping of articular surfaces to remove irregularities (osteophytes) and erosions. It can be performed as an isolated procedure or in conjunction with meniscal repair. It appears to be more suited for small, isolated areas of disease, as opposed to the practice of removing 3–4 mm of the entire anterior-superior slope of the condyle. Follow-up of condyloplasty patients shows significant evidence of progressive degeneration with sclerosis and erosion. Fibrocartilage does not regenerate in areas where condyloplasty has been performed. Because of this, this procedure in isolation or in conjunction with meniscular surgery has largely been abandoned.

Eminoplasty

Eminoplasty can be an important adjunct in the surgical correction of internal derangements, or it can be used alone for treatment of hypermobility. Standard texts have defined normal maximal translation of the condyle as the point where the greatest convexity of the condyle meets the greatest convexity of the articular eminence. In practice, as many as 60% of normal subjects translate more anterior than that point without any symptoms. Subluxation occurs when the condyle translates anterior to its normal range and the patient exhibits a temporary locking or "sticking" sensation that either abates spontaneously or can be reduced with manual self-manipulation. Dislocation is a more severe hypertranslation where the condyle locks out anterior to the eminence to a position where it cannot be self-reduced. Recurrent dislocation is treated with eminoplasty. The eminence should be recontoured as far medially as possible to ensure that adequate bone is removed, though this is controversial and some advocate lateral resection as adequate. Computer tomographic (CT) or magnetic resonance imaging (MRI) images can show the extension of the cancellous bone in the eminence, so care is exercised to prevent intracranial exposure of the temporal lobe. Great care should be taken to protect the meniscus and condylar head

Atlas of Temporomandibular Joint Surgery, Second Edition. Edited by Peter D. Quinn and Eric J. Granquist.
© 2015 John Wiley & Sons, Inc. Published 2015 by John Wiley & Sons, Inc.
Companion Website: www.wiley.com/go/quinn/atlasTMJsurgery

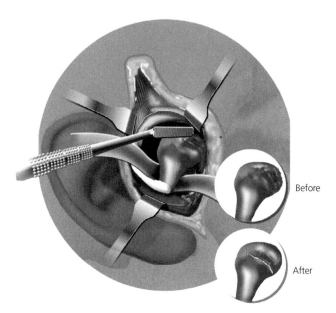

Figure 5.1 Bone file used to contour the head of the condyle during condyloplasty procedure. Although this maneuver can sometimes be beneficial in judiciously removing osteophytes, the fibrocartilage damaged during the procedure does not regenerate and further degenerative changes can occur secondary to the procedure itself.

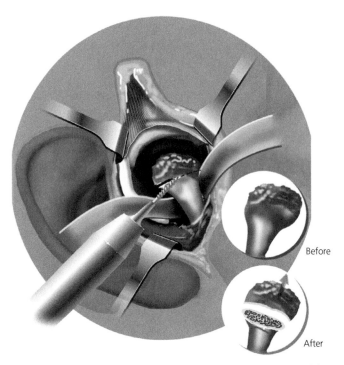

Figure 5.2 High condylar shave. A 1-mm bur is used to remove a 3–4 mm section of the anterior–superior slope of the condyle. The cortical edges are then smoothed with a bone file. This maneuver most often exposes underlying marrow in the condylar head and leads to progressive sclerosis and degeneration.

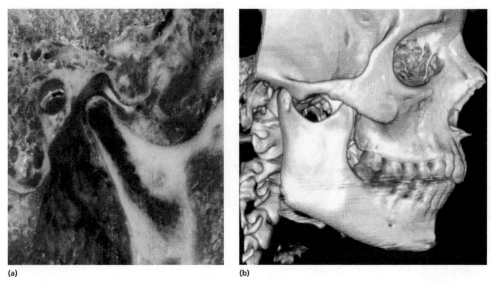

Figure 5.3 (a) Cryosection showing normal appearing condylar head and glenoid fossa. Note the dimensions of the anterior–superior condylar head and its relationship to the posterior aspect of the articular eminence of the glenoid fossa. (b) 3-D CT reconstruction of a normal condyle and glenoid fossa relationship.

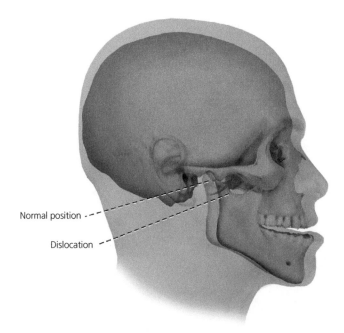

Figure 5.4 Side view of a skull depicting the position of the condyle anterior to the eminence in dislocation. Dislocation implies complete separation of the articular surfaces of the condyle and articular eminence and is nonreducing. Subluxation is partial separation of these surfaces and is self-reducing. In unilateral dislocation, there should be deviation of the midline to the contralateral side with an ipsilateral open bite.

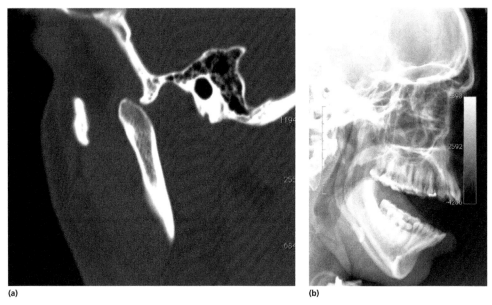

(a)   (b)

Figure 5.5 (a) Sagittal view of a CT scan showing a dislocated temporomandibular joint. Note the anterior-superior position of the condylar head in relation to the articular eminence of the glenoid fossa. (b) Lateral skull film of a patient with bilateral dislocated temporomandibular joints. Note the anterior open bite and pseudo-class-3 relationship.

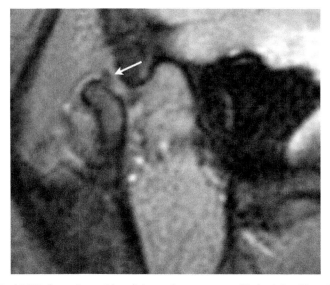

Figure 5.6 A sagittal MRI of a patient with a dislocated temporomandibular joint. Note the anterior band of the meniscus is in a distal position relative to the condylar head (arrow). Image courtesy of Dr. Gerhard Undt.

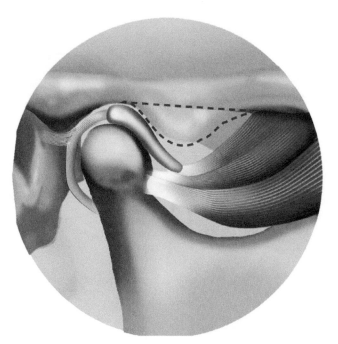

Figure 5.7 Glenoid fossa with eminence reduced. The dotted line denotes the amount of bone removed during the eminoplasty procedure. Note that theoretically the procedure affords greater freedom of movement to the articular disk and lessens the chance of dislocation.

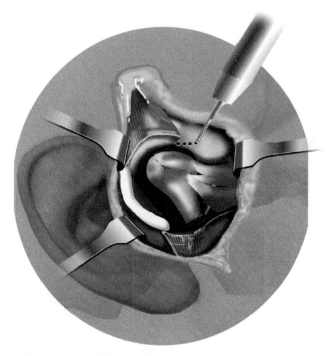

Figure 5.8 Initiating the osteotomy of the articular eminence with a 1-mm fissure bur. Approximately 90% of the cut is performed with the bur.

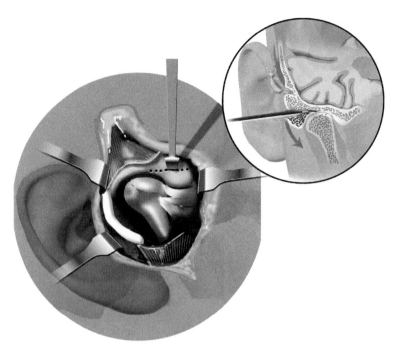

Figure 5.9 The eminoplasty is completed with the aid of an osteotome. The osteotome should be angled inferiorly to ensure the bony cut stays below the base of the skull (see inset).

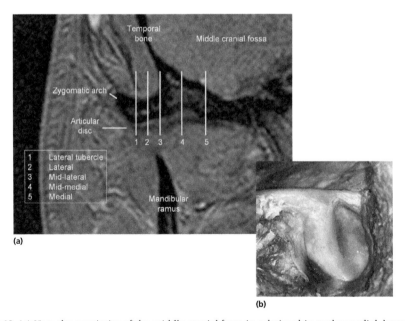

Figure 5.10 (a) Note the proximity of the middle cranial fossa in relationship to the medial–lateral position of the articular eminence. Image courtesy of Dr. Gerhard Undt. (b) Inferior view of cadaver specimen showing medio-lateral extension of articular eminence.

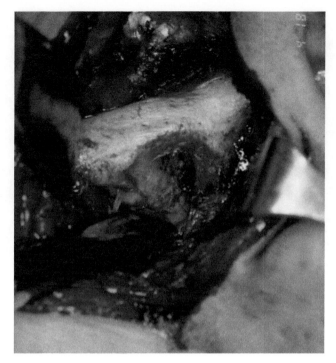

Figure 5.11 Inferior-lateral view of articular eminence showing medial extent (Left Joint).

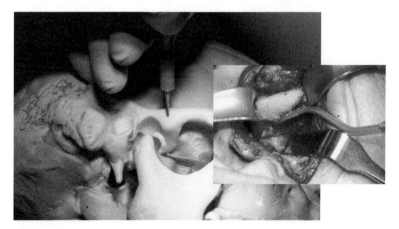

Figure 5.12 Fissure bur positioned for lateral cortical eminoplasty. Alternatively, a reciprocating rasp may be used to reduce the eminence (inset) with less risk of base of skull fracture.

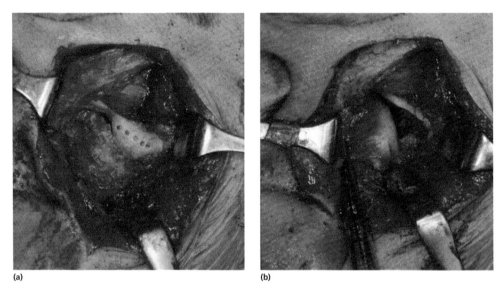

(a)   (b)

Figure 5.13 (a) Bony perforations placed in the articular eminence with a 1-mm Fisher bur to outline the articular eminoplasty. (b) Status post eminoplasty. Reduction of the eminence is required to ensure an unobstructed path of condylar translation.

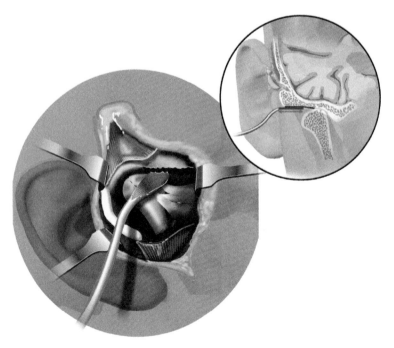

Figure 5.14 A reciprocating rasp may be used to perform the eminoplasty. Great care should be taken to avoid perforation into the middle cranial fossa (inset).

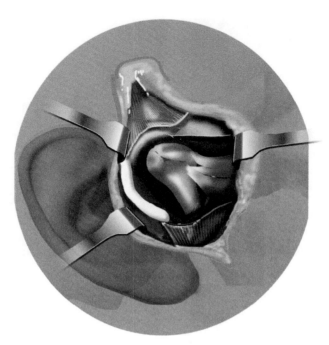

Figure 5.15 After eminoplasty is complete, the mandible is manipulated intraoperatively to ensure unobstructed condylar motion during normal range of motion without dislocation.

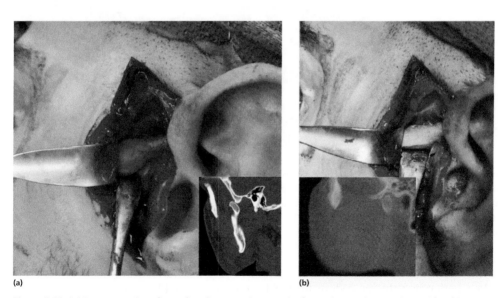

(a)   (b)

Figure 5.16 (a) Intraoperative photo showing prominent articular eminence in a patient with a history of persistent dislocation requiring emergency room intervention for reduction of the condyle. Inset showing CT of the same patient with the condyle dislocated. (b) Same patient following eminoplasty performed with a rasp. A Seldon retractor is placed during the procedure to protect the meniscus. Inset shows the postoperative cone beam CT with near complete reduction of the eminence, which will allow for unobstructed movement of the condyle.

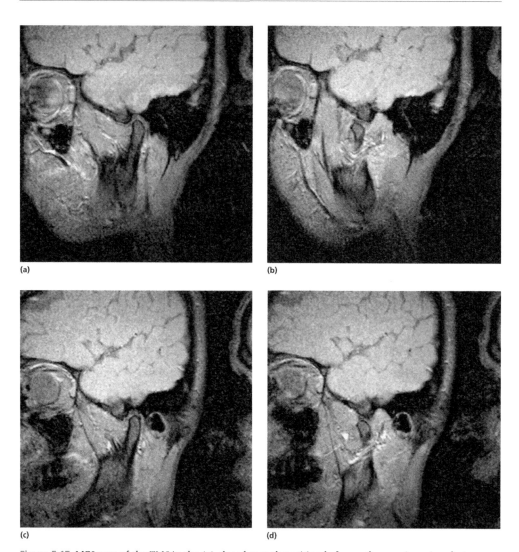

Figure 5.17 MRI scan of the TMJ in the (a) closed-mouth position before arthroscopic eminoplasty and (b) open-mouth position before arthroscopic eminoplasty. MRI scan of a left TMJ (c) in the closed-mouth position 12 months after arthroscopic eminoplasty and (d) open-mouth position 12 months after arthroscopic eminoplasty. The translation of the condyle is slightly limited. Image courtesy of Dr. Gerhard Undt.

when performing this procedure to avoid iatrogenic degeneration of the condyle. Many surgeons advocate a brief period of intermaxillary fixation to induce joint scarring and minimize translation of the condyle, but care should be taken when employing this technique to avoid inadvertent ankylosis of the joint. Finally, some surgeons advocate the need to perform this procedure bilaterally in order to minimize recurrence.

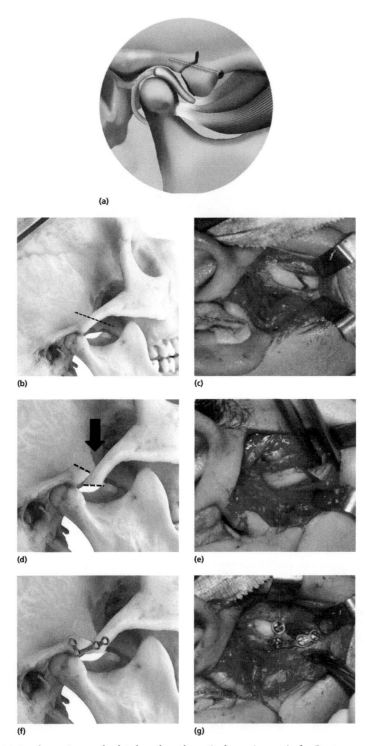

Figure 5.18 (a) An alternative method to lengthen the articular eminence is the Dautrey procedure, in which the zygomatic arch is osteotomized and then fractured in an inferior position. It is subsequently secured to the depth of the articular eminence to lengthen the slope of the posterior eminence. (b and c) Skull model and intraoperative imaging showing osteotomy position (dashed line). (d and e) Skull model and intraoperative image demonstrating inferior repositioning of the distal segment of the zygomatic arch. (f and g) Skull model and intraoperative imaging with distal segment secured in place with hardware. The distal portion of the zygoma now functions to mechanically block anterior dislocation of the condyle. (Images (b) to (g) are the courtesy of Dr. Paul Henrique Luiz de Freital)

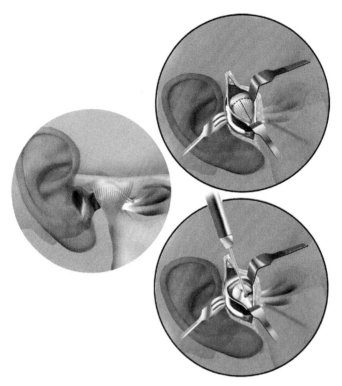

Figure 5.19 Condylectomy is performed through the standard endaural approach used to identify the neck of the condyle at the level of the sigmoid notch below the most inferior-lateral capsular attachment. The condyle is sectioned while protection is provided to the interior maxillary artery, which lies medial to the condylar neck. In the high condylectomy, 7–8 mm of the entire condylar head is removed for intractable temporomandibular joint pain that is unresponsive to medical therapy. This differs from condylectomy performed for prosthetic joint replacement or costochondral rib grafting, in which the osteotomy cut is at the base of the coronoid to prevent postsurgical ankylosis.

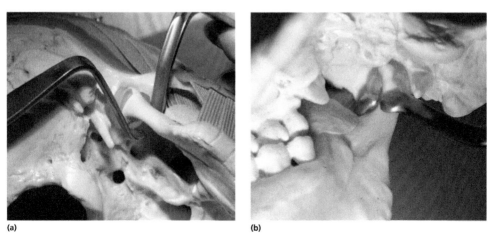

(a)   (b)

Figure 5.20 (a and b) Dunn-Dautrey retractors in place for condylectomy. These retractors protect the internal maxillary artery during the osteotomy.

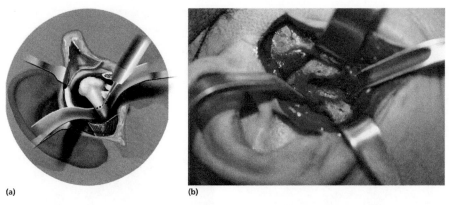

(a)   (b)

Figure 5.21 (a) One millimeter fissure bur is used to make the osteotomy cut at the neck of the condyle. (b) Intraoperative photo showing proper placement of the Dunn-Dautrey retractors prior to the osteotomy in order to ensure protection of the internal maxillary artery.

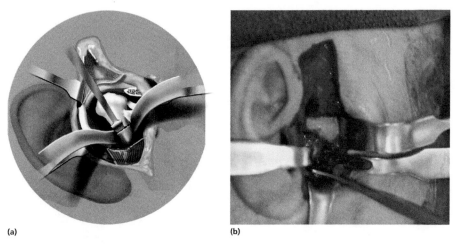

(a)   (b)

Figure 5.22 (a and b) Diagram and photo showing placement of small T-bar osteotome. A mallet is used to gently tap and separate the remaining medial cortex of the condylar neck.

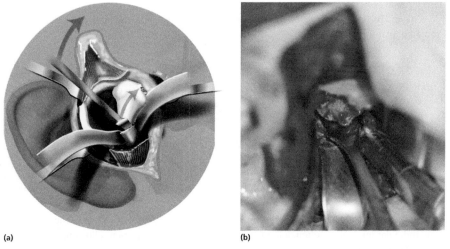

(a)   (b)

Figure 5.23 (a and b) Diagram and photo showing the T-bar osteotome rotated 90° in order to mobilize the condylar head.

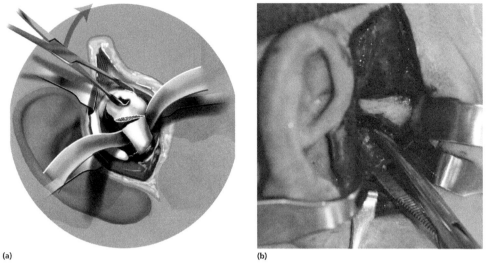

(a)

(b)

Figure 5.24 (a and b) Diagram and photo showing the use of a bone-holding forceps used to carefully remove the condylar head. A sharp periosteal elevator is often used to strip the lateral pterygoid attachment from the anterior surface of the condylar neck (fovea).

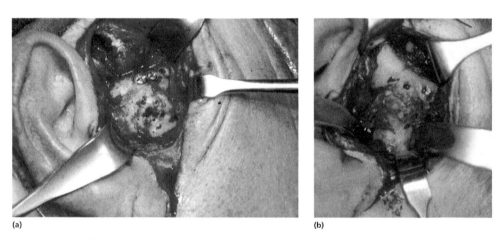

(a)

(b)

Figure 5.25 (a and b) Intraoperative images showing extensive posttraumatic bony ankylosis of the temporomandibular joint.

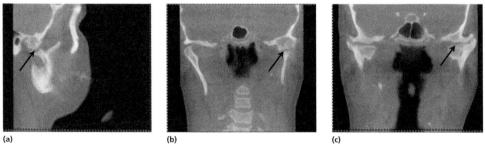

(a)

(b)

(c)

Figure 5.26 (a) Lateral and coronal (b and c) cone beam CT showing bony ankylosis of the temporomandibular joint. Note, often, a pseudarthrosis (arrow) will be present allowing for up to 10 mm of jaw movement.

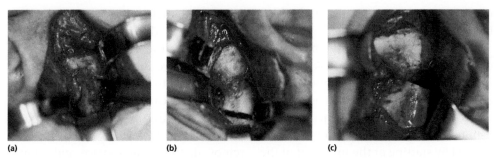

(a)   (b)   (c)

Figure 5.27 Series showing sequence of osteotomies for a condylectomy involving an ankylosed joint (a). Initial osteotomy should be made away from the ankylosed mass often at the level of the condylar neck (b). This avoids unwanted fracture into the skull base or entrance into the middle cranial fossa. Once the ankylosis is freed inferiorly, the condyle can then be safely removed via the pseudarthrosis. (c) Status post condylectomy, with additional bone removed as necessary via superior repositioning of the condyle into the empty glenoid fossa.

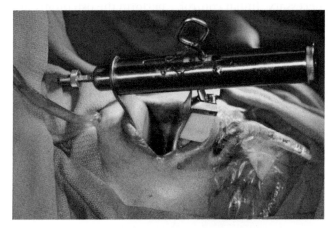

Figure 5.28 Use of a spring-loaded Bell exerciser to lyse adhesions status-post condylectomy.

Condylectomy

As an isolated procedure for joint pain, condylectomy has been largely abandoned. It is a necessary surgical maneuver to treat ankylosis and/or prepare the joint for a total alloplastic prosthesis or a costochondral graft. The procedure involves a standard preauricular approach with special emphasis on visualizing the base of the condylar neck at the level of the sigmoid notch.

Many surgeons also complete the inferior dissection through a modified posterior mandibular incision before the condylectomy. This procedure allows digital access to the medial surface of the ramus (from below) to apply pressure to the internal maxillary artery in the event it is severed while the condyle is sectioned. Because of the proximity of the artery to the condylar neck, specially designed retractors (e.g., Dunn-Dautrey condylar retractors) should be placed before the osteotomy.

A two-step osteotomy has been developed to minimize risk to the internal maxillary artery and ensure adequate bone removal if a total joint replacement will be performed. With a 1-mm fissure bur, an osteotomy is performed by starting at the midpoint of the condylar neck, sparing the medial cortex. A T-bar osteotome is gently tapped and torqued to complete the condylar cut. If bleeding occurs, the cut must be quickly completed to allow access to the area for adequate compression and ligation, if this measure is necessary. Initial control can be maintained with thrombin-soaked sponges, Avitene (collagen), or Flowseal. Pressure and medium Hemoclips can be used if the severed vessel can be visualized. As previously

mentioned, digital compression can also be applied to the medial aspect of the ramus from the retromandibular incision. The retromandibular incision also allows access to the superior branches of the external carotid artery if ligation is required in case of severe hemorrhage (see Chapter 11). Once the condyle is removed, this creates space and allows the surgeon to superiorly reposition the ramus. This allows easier access to the second step of the osteotomy and places this bone cut away from the internal maxillary artery. This maneuvers also allows the surgeon to easily and safely perform the osteotomy at the level of the sigmoid notch, while also decreasing the risk of injury to the facial nerve.

In cases of ankylosis, sectioning the condyle at a level below the ankylosis (usually at the sigmoid notch)

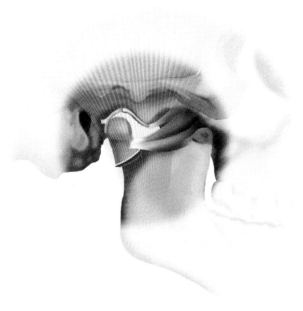

Figure 5.29 Ward condylotomy. Note the telescoping of the condylar segment in an anterior and inferior position. This malpositioned condyle would theoretically unload the meniscus and result in a more physiologic condyle-disk position.

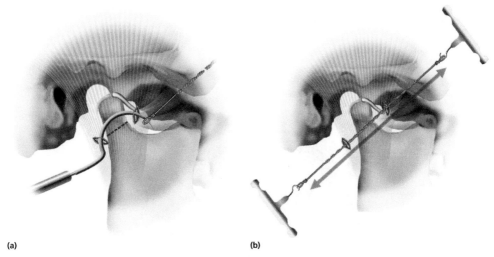

(a)   (b)

Figure 5.30 (a) Ward condylotomy. Costich needle is passed posterior to the ramus with the exit point in the coronoid notch. Great care is taken to ensure the needle is passed in close proximity to the lateral surface of the condylar neck to avoid entrapping the internal maxillary artery between the Gigli saw and the condylar neck. (b) Carefully sectioning the condylar neck at the level of the sigmoid notch, the operator does not bring the Gigli saw completely through all the cortical bone and periosteum on the lateral side but rather leaves a small bridge of bone and soft tissue that can be fractured with digital pressure. This prevents a complete dislocation of the condylar segment out of the glenoid fossa by the unopposed lateral pterygoid muscle.

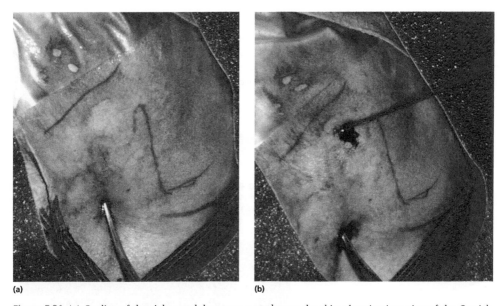

(a)   (b)

Figure 5.31 (a) Outline of the right condyle ramus complex on the skin, showing insertion of the Costich needle with entry posterior to the posterior border of the mandible. This technique was designed to bring the sharp tip of the needle directly behind the neck of the condyle and cause the tip of the needle to exit through the coronoid notch. Care must be taken during this maneuver to remain lateral to the internal maxillary artery. (b) Costich needle exiting through the coronoid notch with Gigli saw attached to the perforation in the terminal tip of the needle. The Gigli saw is then pulled back through the coronoid incision so that its cutting surface lies along the medial surface of the condylar neck.

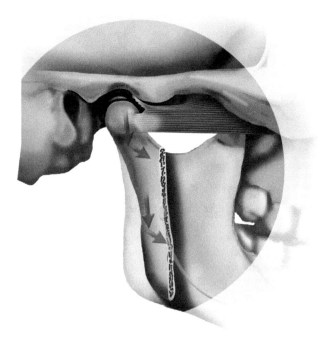

Figure 5.32 Compared with the Ward condylotomy, vertical subcondylar osteotomy offers a more controlled approach to condylar repositioning. In this intra-oral osteotomy procedure, the surgeon is able to attain a more controlled vector of condylar positioning and maximize bone-to-bone contact between the distal and proximal fragments. This procedure also poses less risk for a total dislocation of the condylar head from the glenoid fossa, which can occur with the Ward condylotomy.

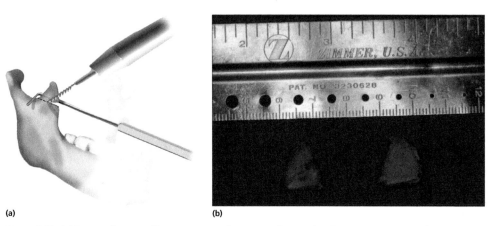

(a)   (b)

Figure 5.33 (a) Intraoral coronoidectomy. Note placement of nerve hook to ensure proper placement of the fissure bur. An osteotomy placed too low along the ramus may result in a condylar fracture. (b) Coronoid fragments after coronoidectomy.

is recommended before attempting to separate the ankylotic bone at the superior glenoid fossa margin. This minimizes iatrogenic entry into the middle cranial fossa.

Condylotomy

Condylotomy for chronic temporomandibular joint pain was popularized by Ward in 1952. Initially performed with a Gigli saw, the procedure was designed to induce a displaced fracture through the condylar neck so that the condyle would be repositioned inferiorly and anteriorly. This would allow the condylar head to seat under the displaced meniscus and unload the posterior attachment.

Nickerson, Hall, and others have renewed interest in the concept of this procedure, and they have popularized an open approach to the condylotomy. An intraoral, subsigmoid, vertical osteotomy is performed, and the patient is maintained in intermaxillary fixation with elastics for a 2- to 4-week period. Unlike the intra-oral vertical ramus osteotomy for orthognathic surgery, the periosteum along the medial and lateral aspect to the inferior border is elevated to achieve condylar sag. The proximal segment should be placed lateral to the distal segment in order to avoid medial displacement of the condyle. The success of this procedure for osteoarthritis and internal derangement appears to be associated with the degree of increased joint space achieved. Condylotomy has the advantage of minimizing damage to the articular and meniscal structures inherent in open arthroplasty and decreasing the potential formation of intra-articular adhesions. Risk of neurovascular injury, malocclusion, and the need for a period of IMF are the primary disadvantages of this procedure.

Further reading

Cherry CQ, Frew A. (1977) High condylectomy for treatment of arthritis of the temporomandibular joint. *J Oral Surg*, 35:285.

Courtemanche AD, Son-Hing QR. (1979) Eminectomy for chronic recurring subluxation of the temporomandibular joint. *Ann Plast Surg*, 3:23.

Dunn MJ. *et al.* (1981) Temporomandibular joint condylectomy: a technique and postoperative follow-up. *Oral Surg Oral Med Oral Path*, 51:363.

Granquist EJ, Quinn PD. (2011) Total reconstruction of the temporomandibular joint with a stock prosthesis. *Atlas Oral Maxillofac Surg Clin North Am*, 19:221.

Lawlor MG. (1982) Recurrent dislocation of the mandible: treatment of ten cases by the Dautrey procedure. *Br J Oral Surg*, 20:14.

Sanders B. (1980) An evaluation of the temporomandibular eminence reduction as a treatment for recurrent dislocation and chronic subluxation: the potential benefits versus the anatomical hazard. *Oral Health*, 70:30.

Undt G. (2011) Temporomandibular joint eminectomy for recurrent dislocation. *Atlas Oral Maxillofac Surg Clin North Am*, 19:189.

Westesson P-L. (1985) Structural hard-tissue changes in temporomandibular joints with internal derangement. *Oral Surg Oral Med Oral Pathol*, 59:220.

Westesson P-L, Rohlin M. (1984) Internal derangement related to osteoarthrosis in temporomandibular joint autopsy specimens. *Oral Surg Oral Med Oral Pathol*, 57:17.

CHAPTER 6

Trauma

Facial injuries are increasingly common in modern society. This increase can be attributed to technologic development of faster automobiles and other modes of transportation, in addition to increased hostility among drivers and a rise in assaults and other forms of interpersonal violence. The temporomandibular joint is certainly not exempt from injury related to these factors. The anatomic complexity of this region makes diagnosis and treatment particularly challenging. Additionally, the role of the temporomandibular joint in the functional processes of speech, mastication, swallowing, and facial expression makes proper management of these injuries paramount. Few areas of oral and maxillofacial surgery have generated as much controversy as the management of injury to the temporomandibular region. This chapter reviews current methods of evaluation, diagnosis, and management of injuries to this region. Pertinent anatomic review and approaches to the temporomandibular joint can be found in Chapter 3.

Incidence, etiology, and pattern of fracture

The literature reports variable statistics for the incidence of fracture involving the mandibular condyle. Early studies report the incidence of mandibular fractures to be as low as 8%, with later reports as high as 50%. The relatively low incidence in early studies may relate to differences in the way fractures were reported, but they probably result from advances in the field of diagnostic imaging, which now allows more accurate detection of these fractures. A reasonable assumption is that fractures involving the condylar process probably compose between one-quarter and one-third of all mandibular fractures.

The type of fracture produced by an injury depends partly on the age of the patient and the magnitude and direction of the force. However, certain mechanisms of injury consistently result in specific fracture patterns. Therefore, knowledge of the mechanism of injury may yield clues to guide the clinician

Atlas of Temporomandibular Joint Surgery, Second Edition. Edited by Peter D. Quinn and Eric J. Granquist.
© 2015 John Wiley & Sons, Inc. Published 2015 by John Wiley & Sons, Inc.
Companion Website: www.wiley.com/go/quinn/atlasTMJsurgery

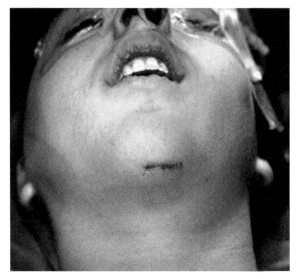

Figure 6.1 Fifteen-year-old with a submental laceration that had been closed 72 h earlier. No intraoral exam had been performed, and the condylar fracture was undiagnosed. Trauma in the submental and symphyseal region should always raise suspicion for a mandibular condylar fracture.

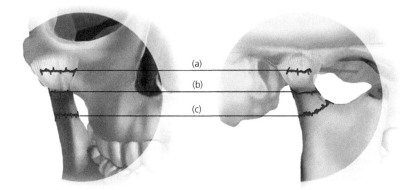

Figure 6.2 Diagram of the levels of condylar fractures. (a) Intracapsular (or condylar head) fracture, (b) condylar neck fracture, and (c) subcondylar fracture.

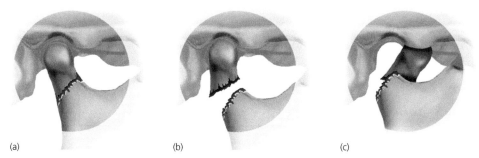

Figure 6.3 Relationship of the condylar (proximal) segment to the mandibular (distal) segment.
(a) Nondisplaced. Normal relationship of the condylar head to the glenoid fossa. (b) Displaced. Condylar head remains within the glenoid fossa, but the proximal segment is not aligned with the distal component.
(c) Dislocated. The condylar head rests completely outside the boundaries of the glenoid fossa.

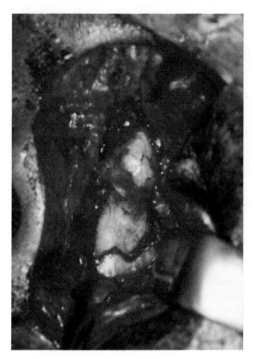

Figure 6.4 Subcondylar fracture. Notice the anterior edge of the fracture begins at the level of the sigmoid notch and courses posteriorly and inferiorly.

during the patient's first visit. For example, a direct blow to the temporomandibular joint region may result in a fracture of the underlying condyle. However, this event is fairly uncommon because of the protection afforded to the condyle by the lateral rim of the glenoid fossa. More commonly, a blow directed horizontally to the mandibular body, such as that delivered by a fist, results in a fracture of the ipsilateral mandibular body and the contralateral condyle. A force delivered to the parasymphyseal region may also cause an ipsilateral condylar fracture. When a force is directed axially to the chin, such as when the chin strikes the ground after a fall or the dashboard during an automobile accident, force is transmitted along the mandibular body to the condyles. This typically results in a symphyseal or parasymphyseal fracture combined with a unilateral or bilateral fracture of the condylar region. When the condyles are driven superiorly and posteriorly into the glenoid fossa, concomitant fracture of the tympanic plate with damage to the

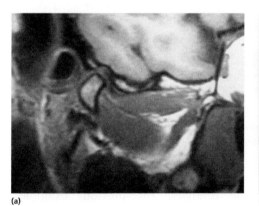

(a)

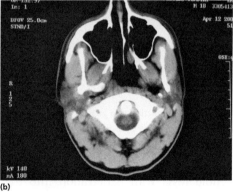

(b)

Figure 6.5 (a) MRI depicting the anterior-medial pull of the lateral pterygoid muscle. (b) Dislocated subcondylar fracture with the proximal segment located anterior and medial along the direction of pull of the lateral pterygoid.

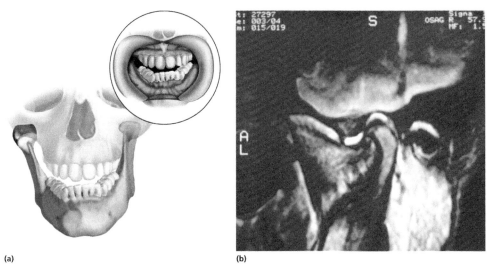

(a)   **(b)**

Figure 6.6 (a) Hemarthrosis. Contusion of the temporomandibular joint should be suspected when a new posterior open bite (inset) without evidence of fracture is seen. Treatment should include early joint mobilization. (b) Sagittal MRI section showing gross effusion in the superior joint space. Note the bright signal of joint effusion and distension of the superior joint space.

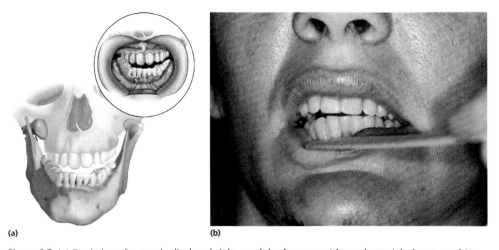

(a)   **(b)**

Figure 6.7 (a) Depiction of a grossly displaced right condylar fracture with resultant right laterognathia and a left open bite (inset). (b) Patient with premature left posterior contact and right posterior open bite.

external auditory canal or fracture of the glenoid fossa with penetration into the middle cranial fossa may result. Because children have a greater modulus of elasticity in bone, a blow to the chin may result in bilateral "green stick" fractures of the condyles. The previous examples demonstrate that the mechanism of injury provides useful insight into the type of injury to be expected.

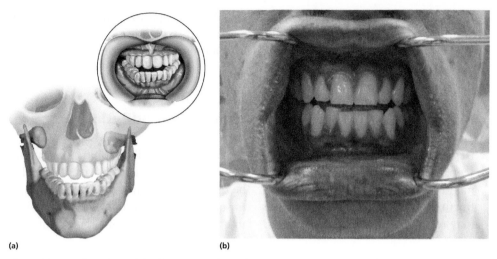

(a)   (b)

Figure 6.8 (a) Bilateral condylar fractures with resultant apertognathia (inset). (b) Patient with new anterior open bite following blunt trauma to his chin. Note the lack of mamelons present on the anterior incisors, this suggesting that the apertognathia is secondary to the trauma and not congenital.

Signs and symptoms associated with condylar fracture

A thorough history of the mechanism of injury should always precede the clinical examination of a patient with a suspected fracture or injury of the mandibular condyle. Patients reporting malocclusion including premature contact or new open bite, difficulty opening, or preauricular pain should raise the suspicion of a condylar fracture. The patient with a fracture of the mandibular condyle usually has a history suggestive of this finding and one or more of the following physical findings:

1 Evidence of facial trauma that may include contusion, abrasion, laceration of the chin, ecchymosis, and hematoma in the temporomandibular region. These injuries should alert the examiner to possible fractures underlying not only the area of injury but also the ipsilateral and contralateral temporomandibular joint.

2 Laceration or bleeding of the external auditory canal. This may result from fracture of the anterior tympanic plate from a posteriorly displaced condyle.

3 Swelling over the temporomandibular joint region may be secondary to hematoma or edema from a fracture.

4 Facial asymmetry. This may be due to foreshortening of the mandibular ramus caused by overlap or telescoping of the proximal and distal fracture segments.

5 Pain and tenderness to palpation over the affected temporomandibular joint.

6 Crepitus over the affected joint. This is caused by the friction of the irregular fracture ends sliding over one another during mandibular movement.

7 Malocclusion. A unilateral condylar fracture usually results in ipsilateral

premature contact of the posterior dentition caused by foreshortening of the ramus on the fracture side. A contralateral posterior open bite is due to canting of the mandible. Bilateral condylar fractures may result in a marked anterior open bite and retrognathia.

8 Deviation of the mandible may be seen at rest or on opening. The mandible may deviate to the side of fracture. Bilateral condylar fractures may result in little midline deviation.

9 Muscle spasms with associated trismus and pain.

10 Dentoalveolar injuries are apparent.

Imaging of the temporomandibular region

Maxillofacial radiographic technique mandates that at least two radiographs be obtained at right angles to each other for adequate evaluation of the temporomandibular joint region. Historically, in

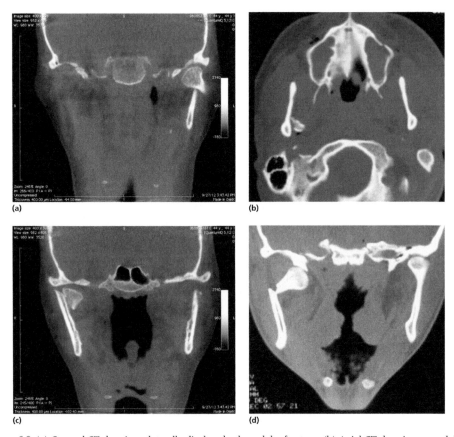

Figure 6.9 (a) Coronal CT showing a laterally displaced subcondylar fracture. (b) Axial CT showing a condylar head fracture with anterior-medial displacement. (c) Coronal CT with a sagittal condylar head fracture with inferior-medial displacement (telescoping). (d) Subcondylar fracture with dislocation of the condylar head.

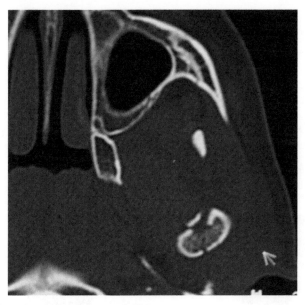

Figure 6.10 Axial CT showing an intracapsular fracture.

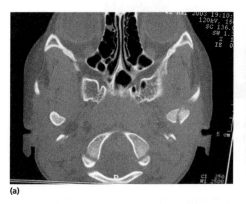
(a)

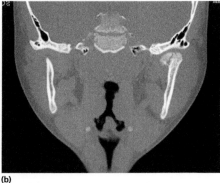
(b)

Figure 6.11 (a) Axial and (b) coronal CT showing minimally displaced condylar head fracture. This type of fracture should be treated with closed reduction for approximately 2 weeks with early mobilization to prevent ankylosis.

most centers the mandible series consists of a posterior–anterior skull image, two lateral oblique views, and a Towne's projection. The panoramic radiograph alone may be a more useful screening tool, with a reported accuracy rate of 92% in detecting all types of mandibular fractures. (The standard mandibular series has an accuracy rate of only 66%.) Unfortunately, many hospital emergency rooms do not have this capability.

With the advent of newer imaging techniques such as computed tomography (CT) and magnetic resonance imaging

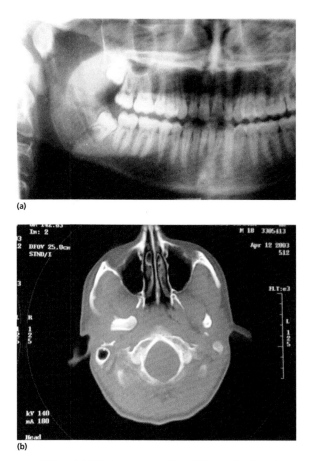
(a)

(b)

Figure 6.12 (a) Panorex and (b) axial CT of a patient with a dislocated right subcondylar fracture. Advanced imaging is often necessary for improved diagnosis and surgical planning in the temporomandibular joint injuries.

(MRI), the standard mandibular and facial survey has been largely supplanted in the diagnosis of maxillofacial trauma. Particularly in trauma centers, where many patients may already require CT imaging, it is often more easier to continue scanning through the facial skeleton. The CT scan yields excellent bony detail of the facial skeleton in multiple views as well as in 3D reconstruction. MRI yields excellent soft tissue detail but less bony resolution when compared with CT

scanning and is rarely obtained, or necessary, in the acute trauma setting.

Classification of fracture of the mandibular condyle

Because condylar fractures are complex with respect to mechanism, anatomy, and associated injuries, development of an all-inclusive classification system for these injuries is difficult at best. Several

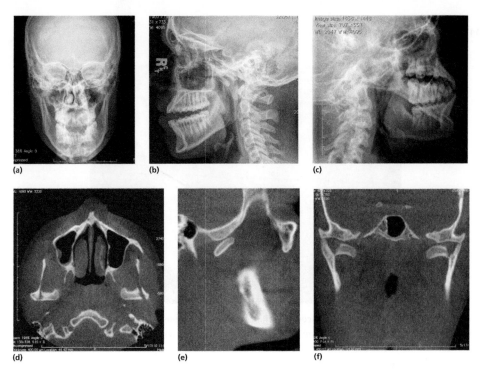

Figure 6.13 (a) PA, (b) lateral, and (c) lateral oblique skull films of a patient seen in the emergency room following trauma to the chin with an anterior open bite. The images were read as normal. (d) Axial, (e) lateral, (f) and coronal CT of the same patient 1 week later. Note the dislocated bilateral subcondylar fractures. Plain films can often be difficult to interpret in the temporomandibular region secondary to overlapping adjacent anatomy.

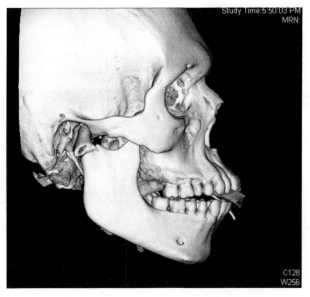

Figure 6.14 3D reconstruction of a severely displaced subcondylar fracture. 3D reconstruction can be utilized to improve visualization of the fracture segment. Subcondylar fractures, below the level of the coronoid notch, are best approached through a retromandibular incision or with a combine preauricular and retromandibular approach.

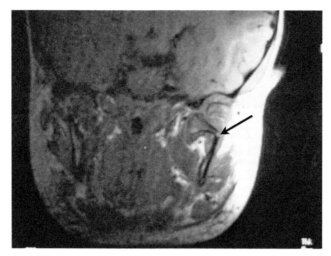

Figure 6.15 MRI depicting gross displacement of a condylar fracture in a 5-year-old girl. Note the complete separation of the cortical plate on the lateral surface (arrow) and the green-sticking of the medial cortical plate. The meniscus can be visualized in a relatively normal position. This fracture was manually reduced via an intraoral approach.

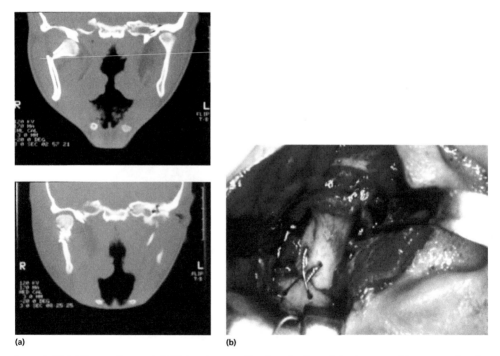

(a)   (b)

Figure 6.16 (a) Pre- and postaxial CT showing a well-reduced subcondylar fracture. (b) "Figure-of-eight" wiring technique used historically to stabilize the fracture segments.

authors have proposed systems based on the anatomic location of the fracture and the relationship of the condylar fragment to the mandible and glenoid fossa. Some of the more comprehensive systems are unsuited to clinical use but warranted for statistical purposes. The lack of consensus regarding classification renders comparison of clinic outcomes research difficult.

In 1977, Lindahl proposed a system that classified condylar fractures based on several factors, including the following: (i) the anatomic location of the fracture, (ii) the relationship of the condylar segment to the mandibular segment, and (iii) the relationship of the condylar head to the glenoid fossa. This system requires that radiographs be obtained in at least two views at right angles to each other (see Figures 7.2 and 7.3). In an effort to establish a more clinically useful classification scheme, MacLennan proposed in 1954 a system based on the relationship of the proximal and distal fracture segments:

Type I Fracture (nondisplaced)

Type II Fracture (fracture deviation). This describes simple angulation of the fracture segments without overlap or separation. Type II fractures include greenstick fractures, commonly seen in pediatric patients.

Type III Fracture (fracture displacement). This is characterized by overlap of the proximal and distal fracture segments. The overlap can be anterior, posterior, medial, or lateral.

Type IV Fracture (fracture dislocation). The condylar head resides completely outside the confines of the glenoid fossa and joint capsule. The dislocation may be anterior, posterior, medial, or lateral.

Treatment of mandibular condyle fractures

The proper management of the fractured mandibular condyle is among the most controversial topics in maxillofacial trauma, generating a wide variety of opinions and proposed treatment modalities. The commonly accepted goal of treatment is the reestablishment of the pretrauma function of the masticatory system, which typically involves the restoration of the preoperative occlusion and facial symmetry. Unlike fractures of other bones, however, the exact anatomic reapproximation of the fracture segments may not be essential. This has been demonstrated in children in whom a conservatively treated displaced or dislocated condylar fracture heals with a perfectly functional and often morphologically-reconstituted condylar process despite a lack of anatomic reduction. This phenomenon is probably related to the remarkable remodeling capacity of bone in children. A similar tendency exists in older patients, although the results are much less predictable.

Early techniques for the management of condylar fracture included various methods and periods of joint immobilization. This approach was chosen because it produced fairly good results and many surgeons feared exposing the temporomandibular region to surgical complications. Moreover, early methods of internal fixation were clearly not preferable to more conservative methods. As surgical techniques improved and methods of rigid fixation were developed, surgeons became more comfortable with open approaches to the joint. An expanding set

Table 6.1 Open reduction of the fractured mandibular condyle.

Absolute indications	Relative indications
1. Displacement of the condyle into the middle cranial fossa	1. Bilateral condylar fractures in an edentulous patient when splints are unavailable or impossible because of ridge atrophy
2. Inability to obtain adequate occlusion with technique	2. Unilateral or bilateral condylar fractures when intermaxillary fixation is not recommended secondary to medical conditions
3. Lateral extracapsular displacement of the condyle	3. Bilateral fractures associated with comminuted midfacial fractures
4. Invasion of the joint by a foreign body	4. Bilateral fractures associated with other gnathic problems

of indications for open surgical intervention evolved, but the technique continued to stimulate a great deal of debate, which persists today (see Table 6.1).

Closed treatment

Available data overwhelmingly supports the belief that many fractures of the mandibular condyle can be successfully treated through conservative means. The closed management of condylar fracture ranges from observation and prescription of a soft diet to variable periods of immobilization followed by intense physiotherapy. If the patient is able to establish and maintain a normal occlusion with a minimal amount of discomfort, no active treatment may be necessary. The patient should be encouraged to eat soft foods and maintain as near normal function as possible. Close supervision is mandatory, and both clinical and radiographic reevaluation should be performed at the first sign of occlusal instability, deviation with opening, or increasing pain. Those findings may indicate the conversion of a nondisplaced fracture to a displaced one that requires more aggressive treatment. Only responsible patients who are committed to a period of close follow-up should be considered for the observation-only treatment regimen.

Usually the presence of malocclusion, deviation with function, or significant pain necessitates some form of immobilization. This generally involves intermaxillary fixation with arch bars, eyelet wires, or splints. The length of the period of immobilization is controversial: It must be long enough to allow initial union of the fracture segments but short enough to prevent complications such as muscular atrophy, joint hypomobility, and ankylosis. Currently the period of immobilization ranges from 7 to 21 days, with most advocating 14 days of intermaxillary fixation followed by a soft, nonchew diet. This period of immobilization and diet restriction may be increased or decreased depending on concomitant factors such as the age and nutritional status of the patient, the level of the fracture, the degree of displacement, and the presence of additional fractures.

Open reduction of the fractured mandibular condyle

Although incontrovertible evidence to support the efficacy of open techniques is lacking, a specific group of individuals appear to benefit from open surgical intervention. Zide and Kent, Raveh *et al.*, and others have proposed a set of absolute and relative indications for open reduction of the fractured mandibular condyle. However, each case should always be evaluated individually (see Table 6.1).

Once the decision has been made to use an open technique, the next step in treatment planning is to select a surgical approach. Over the years, many approaches to the temporomandibular joint have been developed, including intraoral, pre-auricular, endaural, retroauricular, retro-mandibular, and rhytidectomy approaches. Each has its own advantages, disadvantages, and complications. Many of these approaches have fallen from favor; only the preauricular, submandibular, and intraoral routes are routinely used in most centers. The location of the fracture and the degree of displacement are the prime determinants in the selection of the approach to the joint. If the fracture is intracapsular or high on the condylar neck, the preauricular or endaural approach is preferred. This approach offers better access, greater visibility of the fracture site, ease of manipulating soft tissues within the joints, and relative ease of placement of fixation devices. The inherent disadvantages are the possibility of damage to the facial nerve and the presence of a facial scar. Subcondylar fractures, and fractures located lower in the condylar neck, may be more easily reached by a submandibular or poste-rior-mandibular approach. The danger of this technique is possible injury to the marginal mandibular nerve with subsequent weakness of the depressor muscles of the lower lip. Often, the combination of these approaches is necessary to gain adequate access to reduce and fixate the fracture segments. Several authors have advocated an intraoral approach to fracture of the condyle. This approach allows the sur-geon to visualize the fracture reduction and the occlusion simultaneously, mini-mizes risk of damage to the facial nerve, and prevents an unsightly facial scar. Disadvantages include a more limited access, especially in high subcondylar and condylar neck fractures, and the difficulty of placing fixation devices (see Chapter 3 for additional discussion on approaches).

Methods of fixation for condylar fractures

After the fracture site has been adequately exposed, the segments must be reduced to their preinjury position. In the case of minimal displacement, this reduction is accomplished by using a hemostat or other instrument to manipulate the proximal fragment into position. When the condylar segment is more signifi-cantly displaced or dislocated from the fossa, reduction becomes more difficult. Because of the pull of the lateral pterygoid muscle, the condylar fragment is usually located anterior and medial to the distal segment. Distraction of the mandible in an inferior direction by use of a clamp, towel clip, or stainless steel wire placed at the angle aids in visualizing and manipulating the condylar segment. The condylar segment is then grasped and reduced into its proper location on the mandibular ramus. Stewart and Bowerman suggest inserting a Moule pin into the condyle to assist in positioning this small fragment. Once the fragment is reduced and secured, the pin is removed before wound closure. With severe medial dislo-cation of high condylar fractures that cannot be adequately reduced with other methods, Mikkonen *et al.* and Ellis *et al.*

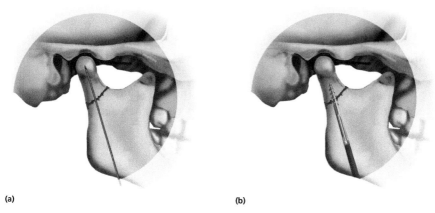

(a)   (b)

Figure 6.17 Various alternative techniques for stabilizing condylar fractures have been described. (a) K-wire placed from an inferior approach through the body of the posterior ramus for reduction of a nondisplaced condylar fracture. (b) Lag-screw-washer technique described by Krenkle. Note the body channel that is drilled to allow perpendicular access to the plane of the fracture for screw access.

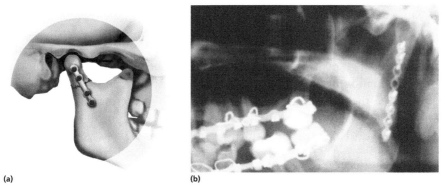

(a)   (b)

Figure 6.18 (a) Rigid fixation of a condylar fracture. Note the presence of at least two screws in the distal and proximal segments. (b) Postoperative panorex showing good reduction with the use of plate fixation.

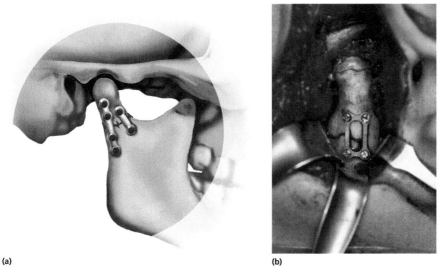

(a)   (b)

Figure 6.19 (a) Often a second plate is required to improve immobilization of the proximal segment. (b) A "square-plate" to place screws horizontally rather than vertically in the proximal and distal segments.

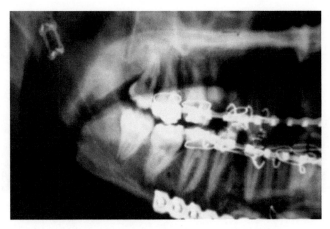

Figure 6.20 Postoperative panorex with a "square" plate configuration in place.

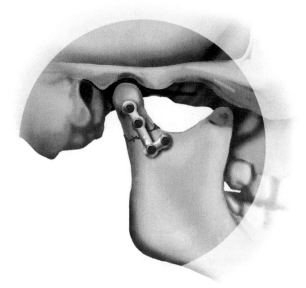

Figure 6.21 Alternative-shaped plates may be utilized to improve rigidity and ensure adequate screw placement with less chance of facial nerve injury.

recommend a submandibular approach for access to perform a vertical ramus osteotomy with subsequent removal of the posterior ramus. This technique allows increased access and visibility to the medially positioned condyle. The surgeon then grasps and removes the condylar fragment while keeping the capsule and disk intact. The posterior ramus and condyle are taken to the back table, where they are placed into proper anatomic relationship and secured obliquely with a 2.0-mm lag screw. The ramus–condyle is then treated as a free

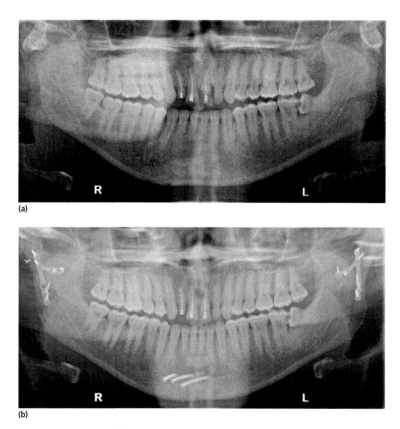

Figure 6.22 (a) Panorex showing bilateral subcondylar fractures. (b) Postoperative image showing well-reduced fractures reduced with a "lamda" plate (Synthes CMF). Images courtesy of Dr. David Stanton.

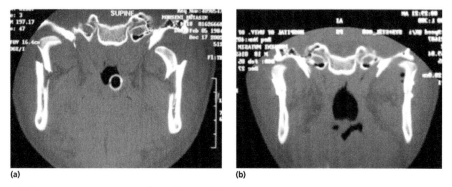

Figure 6.23 (a) Preoperative coronal CT showing bilateral displaced subcondylar fractures.
(b) Postoperative coronal CT showing good reduction and fixation using a four-hole vertical plate.

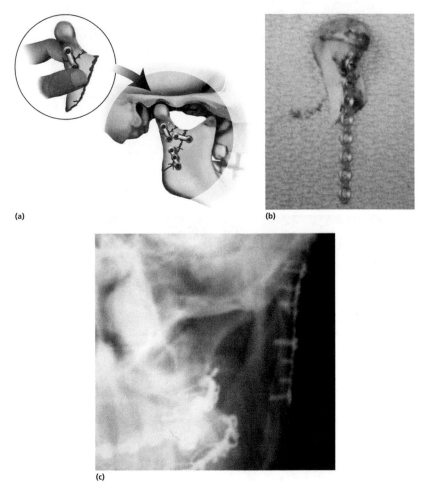

(a)

(b)

(c)

Figure 6.24 (a) Extraoral technique for complicated condylar fracture reduction with completely avulsed condylar segments in complex fracture patterns or fractures that are difficult to visualize or properly reduce. The rigid plate is placed on the proximal fragment and reinserted into the wound through a posterior mandibular incision. (b) This fractured condyle was so grossly displaced from the fossa that it was almost completely severed from its soft tissue attachments. The superior screws were placed extracorporeally, which allowed for improved placement into the small proximal segment. The proximal segment with the plate attached was inserted through a retromandibular incision. (c) Postoperative posterior–anterior showing good reduction and fixation of the fracture.

autogenous bone graft, returned to the field, and secured with two small bone plates. The next step is the selection of a method of fixation to maintain the osteotomy segments in the reduced position.

Historically, a wide variety of fixation techniques have been employed, including suture ligatures, external fixation, K wires, osteosynthesis wires, axial anchor screws, and rigid plates and screws. Because of advances in

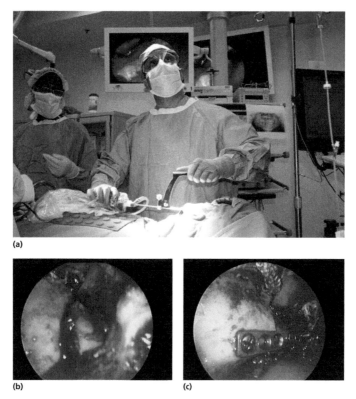

(a)

(b)   (c)

Figure 6.25 (a) Surgeon endoscopically reducing a subcondylar fracture. (b) Endoscopic view of a subcondylar fracture, note lateral and inferior displacement. (c) Endoscopic view following reduction and fixation of the fracture. Image courtesy of Dr. Lee Carrasco.

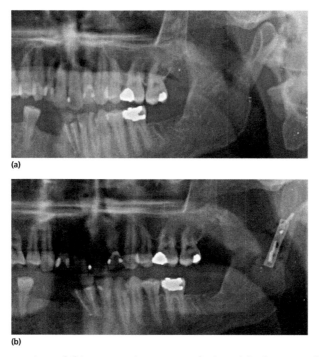

(a)

(b)

Figure 6.26 (a) Preoperative and (b) postoperative panorex of subcondylar fracture reduced and fixated via an endoscopic approach. Image courtesy of Dr. Lee Carrasco.

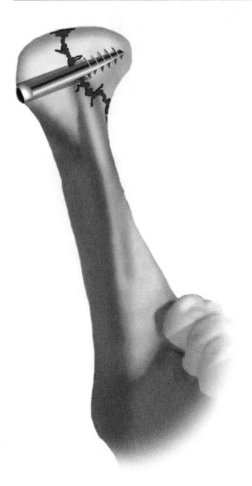

Figure 6.27 Diagram showing lag screw technique for the reduction and fixation of a condylar head fracture.

screw placement in areas where access is difficult and endoscopic techniques have been described. Some surgeons choose not to apply any fixation after reduction of the condyle. This is not advisable because the same muscular pull that caused the initial displacement or dislocation could again cause displacement of the reduced fragment.

Condylar fractures in children

Condylar fractures in children involve mechanisms similar to those of adult injury. However, the incidence of condylar fracture among children is higher, reportedly between 40 and 60% of all mandible fractures. Falls from heights and bicycles are the most common causes of condylar fracture in children, with an incidence of between 30 and 50% of cases. Motor vehicle accidents are second in frequency (26–34%), followed by sports-related injuries (15%) and assault (3%). In most series, boys are affected more than girls by a ratio of 2:1. Carroll *et al.* also noted a seasonal variation in the number of fractures sustained by children; not surprisingly, the increase occurred during the summer months, when children are more active outdoors. Condylar fractures are more difficult to detect in children. First, children with acute injuries are often frightened and intimidated by the busy emergency room and doctors who often are unused to dealing with children. Second, children are less able to convey subjective symptoms of their injuries.

biomaterials, downsizing of hardware, and the availability of instrumentation in most operating rooms, rigid fixation with plates and screws is the most common technique. These plates afford stability in three dimensions, and placement can be accomplished through any of the surgical approaches. Percutaneous trocars have been developed to facilitate accurate

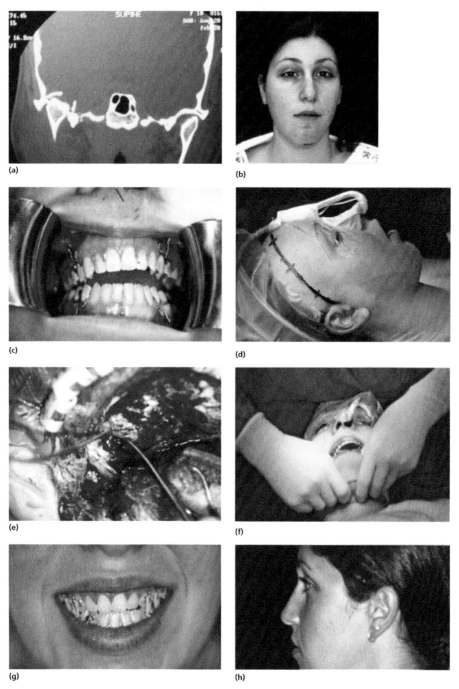

Figure 6.28 (a) Coronal CT showing fracture of the glenoid fossa and condylar head displaced into the middle cranial fossa. (b) Patient preoperative frontal view, note laceration on chin. (c) Preoperative occlusion, note the premature contact and contralateral open bite. (d) Bicoronal incision marked for access to the middle cranial fossa and temporomandibular joint. (e) Neurosurgical exposure prior to condylar reduction is necessary to control any bleeds if they occur and to repair any dural tears. (f) Manual reduction of the displaced condyle. (g) Postoperative image showing intermaxillary fixation. (h) Lateral facial view 6 weeks postoperative. Source: Quinn 1998. Reproduced with permission of Elsevier.

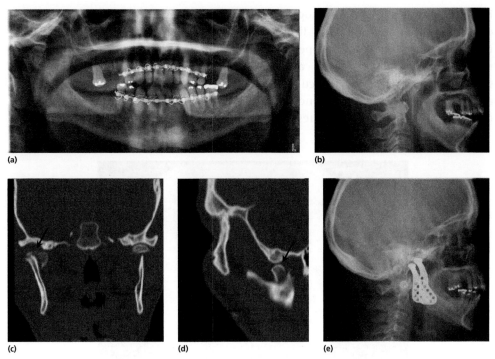

Figure 6.29 (a) Preoperative panorex of patient showing bilateral condylar fractures. (b) Lateral cephalogram of patient, note anterior open bite and premature posterior occlusion. (c) Coronal CT showing bilateral condylar fractures, note comminution of the right condylar head (arrow). (d) Saggital CT showing anterior displacement of the condylar head (arrow) resulting in a mechanic trismus. (e) Lateral cephalogram following bilateral total joint replacement. Note closure of anterior open bite. Image courtesy of Dr. Sotirios Diamantis.

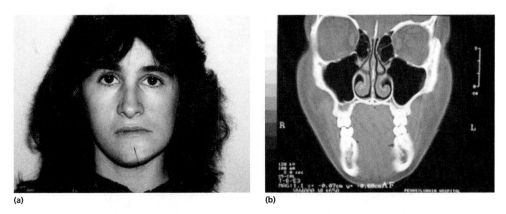

Figure 6.30 (a) A 22-year-old woman who sustained an untreated condylar fracture at 7 years of age. Note the marked left-sided ramus foreshortening with symphyseal asymmetry. (b) Axial CT showing facial asymmetry secondary to untreated condylar fracture. Source: Quinn 1998, figure 6.21a, p. 140. Reproduced with permission of Elsevier.

Finally, physical and radiographic examination is often very difficult. Children are frequently uncooperative, making the detection of an already subtle injury even more difficult. The advent of more rapid CT scanners and the use of sedation techniques have improved the sensitivity of the radiographic examination. The signs and symptoms of condylar fracture in children are similar to those of adults.

Numerous studies have examined the effects of condylar fractures on the masticatory system, growth, and facial

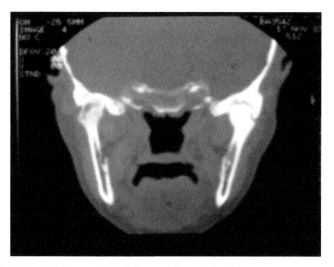

Figure 6.31 Axial CT showing bony ankylosis from a left condylar fracture.

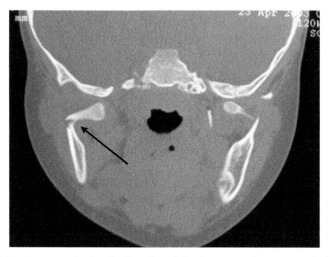

Figure 6.32 Axial CT showing a displaced right subcondylar fracture with "green-stick" fracture of the medial cortex (arrow).

Initial fracture 24 months

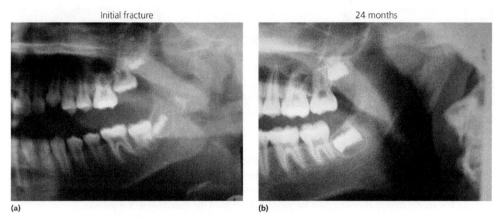

(a)   (b)

Figure 6.33 (a) Pediatric subcondylar fracture treated with closed reduction. (b) Twenty-four months follow-up, note near normal anatomy of the condyle. Image courtesy of Dr. David Stanton.

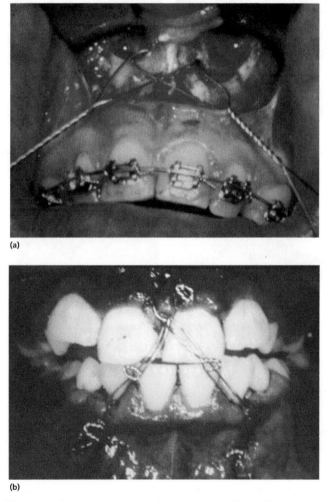

(a)

(b)

Figure 6.34 (a and b) Photos showing anterior nasal spine wire for skeletal fixation of a condylar fracture.

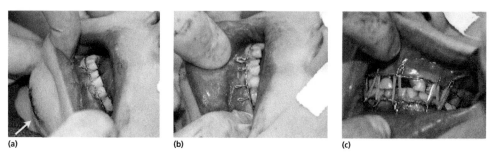

Figure 6.35 (a) Risdon wire can be used for intermaxillary fixation in patients with mixed dentition or with only deciduous teeth. Note the laceration evident in the submental region in this child with a subcondylar fracture (arrow). (b) Once the Risdon wire is in place, interdental ligature can be used to secure the Risdon wire. (c) The secure Risdon wire can then be used for fixation of the mandible to the maxilla.

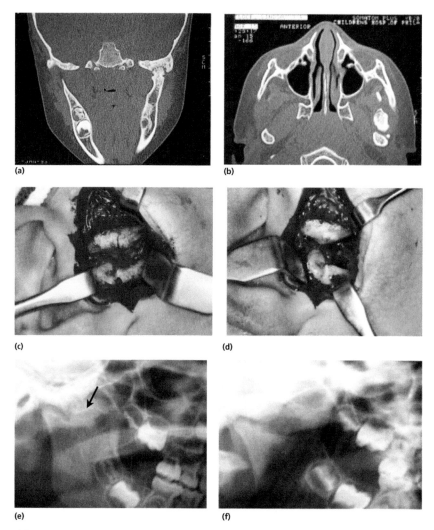

Figure 6.36 (a) Coronal CT of a 5-year-old with an untreated condylar fracture, limited opening, and deviation with opening. (b) Axial CT of the same patient showing displaced condylar head anterior to the condylar stump. (c) Open arthroplastic view showing traumatic ankylosis. (d) Same view showing increased range of motion after removal of the bony obstruction. (e) Preoperative panorex with anterior displaced condylar stump evident (arrow). (f) Postoperative panorex with bony obstruction removed.

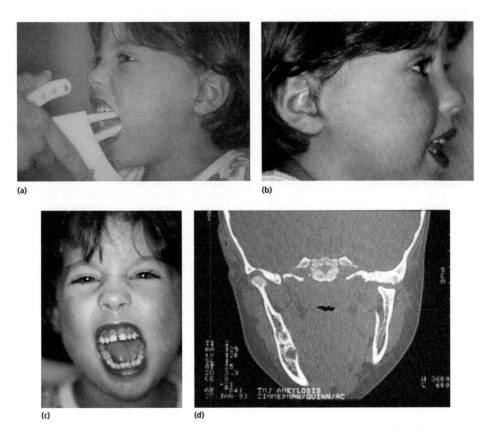

Figure 6.37 (a) Patient from Figure 3.36 undergoing jaw exercise physical therapy. (b) Well-healed endaural incision. (c) Patient demonstrating good jaw function, note slight deviation to the side of the trauma. (d) Postoperative coronal CT demonstrating remodeling of the condylar stump. Source: Quinn 1998, figure 6.53, p. 166. Reproduced with permission of Elsevier.

aesthetics. The Chalmers J. Lyons Academy, MacLennan, Blevins and Gores, Indahl, Lund, and several animal studies conducted by Walker and Boyne are several of the more notable. The conclusions reached by these authors confirm the concept that regardless of the type of injury, the degree of fracture displacement, or the specific treatment used, children have an incredible ability to regenerate a morphologically, anatomically, and functionally normal condylar articulation. Moreover, the younger the individual (up to ~12 years of age), the more complete and rapid the restitution of the condyle. In adolescents, the potential for significant regeneration and remodeling is present but to a lesser degree than in younger children. These authors also overwhelmingly support the use of conservative measures in the treatment of these injuries, with a very brief period of intermaxillary fixation (~7–10 days) being common. This is followed by active movement of the joint, which reduces the formation of scar tissue and prevents ankylosis. These studies also confirm the paucity of clinically significant signs or symptoms of masticatory dysfunction after fracture healing. As with adults (and possibly more important), a closely supervised follow-up program is an absolute requirement because growing children face an increased risk of ankylosis and growth disturbance with resultant facial asymmetry.

Further reading

Chrcanovic BR. *et al.* (2012) 1,454 mandibular fractures: a 3-year study in a hospital in Belo Horizonte, Brazil. *J Cranio-Maxillo-Facial Surg,* 40:116.

Christiansen EL. *et al.* (1987) CT evaluation of trauma to the temporomandibular joint. *J Oral Maxillofac Surg,* 45:920.

Goldberg MH. *et al.* (1971) Auditory canal hemorrhage: a sign of mandibular trauma. *J Oral Surg,* 29:425.

Kent J. *et al.* (1990) Open reduction of fractured mandibular condyles. *Oral Maxillofac Surg Clin North Am,* 2:69.

Oikarinen KS. *et al.* (1991) Signs and symptoms of TMJ dysfunction in patients with mandibular condyle fractures. *Cranio,* 9:58.

Sawazaki R. *et al.* (2010) Incidence and patterns of mandibular condylar fractures. *J Oral Maxillofac Surg,* 68:1252.

Smith DM. *et al.* (2013) 215 mandible fractures in 120 children: demographics, treatment, outcomes, and growth data. *Plast Reconstr Surg,* 131:1348.

Spiessl B. (1989) *Internal fixation of the mandible,* Springer-Verlag, Berlin.

Stewart A, Bowerman JE (1991) A technique for control of the condylar head during open reduction of the mandibular condyle. *Br J Oral Maxillofac Surg,* 29:312.

Zhou H. *et al.* (2013) Changing pattern in the characteristics of maxillofacial fractures. *J Craniofac Surg,* 24:929.

Zide M, Kent J. (1983) Indications for open reduction of mandible condyle fractures. *J Oral Maxillofac Surg,* 41:89.

CHAPTER 7

Autogenous reconstruction of the temporomandibular joint

Autogenous temporomandibular joint (TMJ) reconstruction offers a number of advantages including the potential for growth, biocompatibility, and availability. Autogenous joint replacements, particularly costochondral grafts, are always preferred for the growing patients. The chief disadvantages associated with autogenous grafts are donor-site morbidity and the variability of biologic responses (e.g., resorption, ankylosis, and excessive growth). Autogenous tissues used to reconstruct the TMJ include rib grafts (costochondral), iliac crest, sternoclavicular, and metacarpal joints. Use of costochondral grafts in both pediatric and adult patients has been extensively documented in the literature. The costochondral graft is most adaptable to the TMJ because of its native dimensions. Its cartilaginous cap is composed of hyaline cartilage rather than fibrocartilage, but it appears to withstand the biomechanical stresses of joint function relatively well. It is the preferred method of reconstruction in the pediatric patient. Recently, for patients with large bony and soft tissue defects, distraction osteogenesis has been utilized for reconstruction of the mandible and TMJ. In the adult population, autogenous TMJ reconstruction is largely accomplished with the use of a vascularized bone graft, particularly in patients undergoing tumor resection requiring radiation treatment. Finally, considerable advances continue in the field of tissue engineering and may become a viable option for joint reconstruction in the future.

Costochondral graft

The most widely used autogenous graft for TMJ reconstruction is the costochondral graft and is widely used because of its adaptability, size, and cartilaginous cap. Costochondral grafts can be expected to grow spontaneously in pediatric patients (i.e., those <15 years of age), although this may be problematic and growth is often unpredictable and may result in under- or overgrowth. Ankylosis of costochondral grafts is rare in the pediatric age group but can occur in adult patients, especially those who have undergone multiple operations with extensive fibrosis at the recipient site. In these patients, the risk of heterotopic

Atlas of Temporomandibular Joint Surgery, Second Edition. Edited by Peter D. Quinn and Eric J. Granquist.
© 2015 John Wiley & Sons, Inc. Published 2015 by John Wiley & Sons, Inc.
Companion Website: www.wiley.com/go/quinn/atlasTMJsurgery

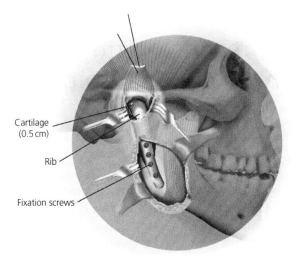

Cartilage
(0.5 cm)

Rib

Fixation screws

Figure 7.1 Diagram showing placement of a costochondral graft for reconstruction of the temporomandibular joint. The graft can be fixated with the use of a plate or screws. Decorticating the graft or the lateral surface of the mandible is unnecessary.

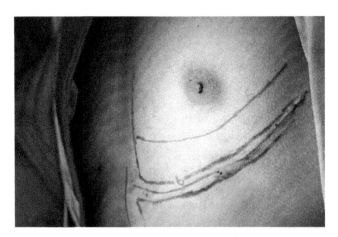

Figure 7.2 A skin marker used to indicate the position of the sixth rib of the contralateral side before harvesting. Note the position to areolar markings. This is of special importance in female patients because an attempt is made to place the incision for the rib harvesting in the inframammary fold.

bone formation is high. In most cases, the contralateral rib is harvested for joint reconstruction.

The ribs most commonly used for joint reconstruction are the fifth, sixth, and seventh ribs. The rib is harvested through a horizontal incision in the inframammary fold. If two ribs are needed, they should be harvested on the same side (e.g., the fourth and sixth ribs or fifth and seventh ribs) to prevent bilateral pneumothorax. Ribs from the ipsilateral side require more contouring because they do not have the ideal

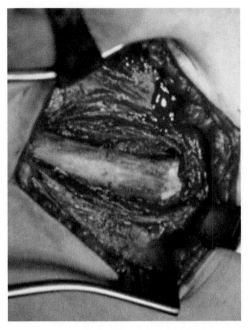

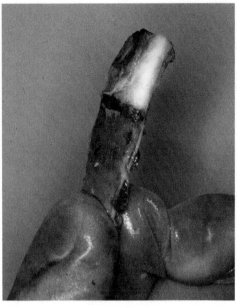

Figure 7.4 Costochondral graft following harvest, with perichondrium intact.

Figure 7.3 Harvesting a rib on the contralateral side, attempt should be made to retain the perichondrium/periosteum over the surface of the periosteum of the cartilage. This helps to reduce the incidence of spontaneous separation at the junction point.

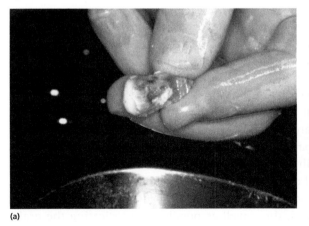

(a)

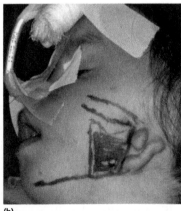

(b)

Figure 7.5 (a) Costochondral graft after the cartilage has been carved to leave a 1-cm cap of cartilage. (b) Patient with hemifacial miscrosomia. Note underdeveloped auricle with inferior position.

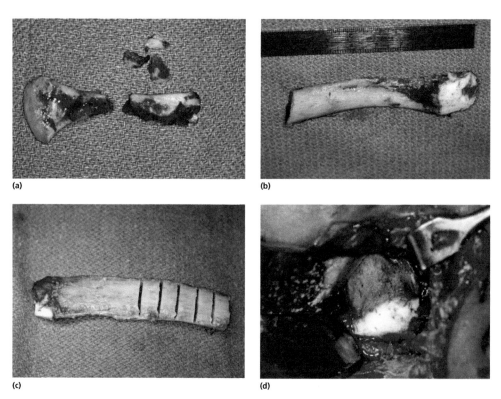

(a)

(b)

(c)

(d)

Figure 7.6 (a) Multiple fragments of an irreparable condylar fracture secondary to bullet wound injury. (b and c) Costochondral graft after harvesting showing scoring the surface to avoid iatrogenic fracture. (d) Endaural incision showing placement of the costochondral graft into the glenoid fossa. Note that the costal cartilage has been contoured with a #15 blade to simulate the shape of the natural condyle. The cartilage is approximately 8–10 mm at its midpoint.

angulation. After dissecting through skin and subcutaneous tissue, the surgeon carefully excises the periosteum on the undersurface of the rib to prevent a pneumothorax. Leaving a strip of periosteum and perichondrium overlying the junction of the rib and the costal cartilage helps prevent separation of the cartilage from the rib during function. Approximately 1 cm of cartilage and 3–4 cm of bone is normally sufficient. After the rib is removed, the wound can be filled with saline and the anesthesiologist can maximally inflate the lungs to look for bubbling in the saline, an initial indication of a pleural tear. Small pleural tears can be closed at that time. An upright chest film should be obtained immediately after surgery to ensure that pneumothorax has not occurred.

Once the rib is harvested, a scalpel blade is used to contour the hyaline cartilage so that it simulates the shape of the condylar head and fits in the fossa as well as possible. Decorticating the graft or the medial surface of the ramus is unnecessary. The graft can be secured to either the lateral ramus or the posterior ramus with circumferential wires, bone screws, or a combination of plates and screws. The surgeon should be careful not to tighten the screws excessively because this can induce a longitudinal fracture in the rib. A small fixation plate is sometimes used with the screws to act as a "washer," dispersing the pressure from the screwheads. The superior–lateral edge of the condylectomy margin should be contoured so that the rib is not displaced laterally by ramal bone. A combination of an endaural incision and a posterior mandibular incision is necessary to properly position and secure the rib graft. Intermaxillary fixation is necessary to allow for initial

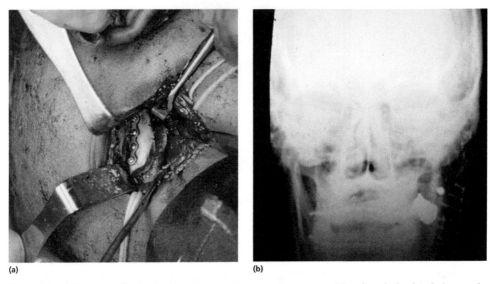

(a)   (b)

Figure 7.7 (a) Retromandibular incision showing the posterior ramus with a four-hole plate being used to fixate the costochondral graft to the lateral ramus. (b) AP skull film showing rigid fixation used and excellent adaptation of the costochondral graft.

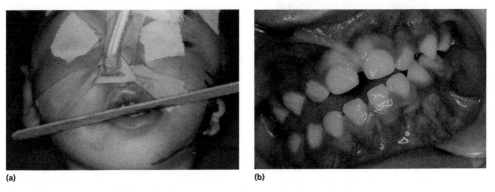

(a)   (b)

Figure 7.8 (a) Patient with hemifacial microsomia. Note occlusal cant (b).

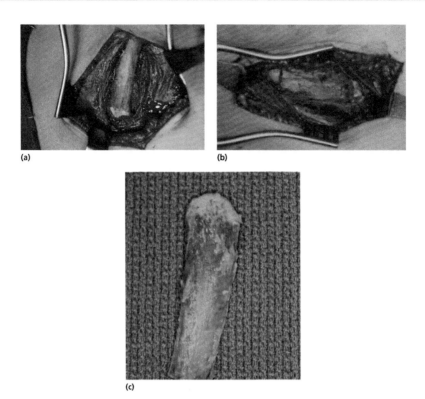

(a)   (b)

(c)

Figure 7.9 (a) Rib exposed prior to harvest. (b) Rib removed, with periosteum intact and no evident air leak. The wound should be flooded with saline and a valsalva maneuver performed to confirm that no air leak exists. If evident, the leak or tear should be repaired or a chest tube placed. (c) Harvested costochondral graft prior to implantation. The cartilagenous cap is approximately 10 mm.

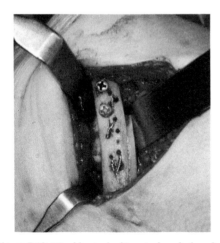

Figure 7.10 "Double-stacked" costochondral graft secured to the lateral border of the ramus with wires and screws.

consolidation of the graft and is usually appropriate for a period of 4–6 weeks. In addition, most clinicians use an acrylic splint that opens the vertical dimension 2–3 mm to prevent early loading of the costochondral graft. Conversely, because prolonged intermaxillary fixation can lead to early ankylosis of the graft, several authors recommend that dermal or temporo-myofascial grafts be used in concert with the costochondral graft.

In the adult patient, particularly with ankylosis, the use of the costochondral graft has limited application when compared to other reconstructive options.

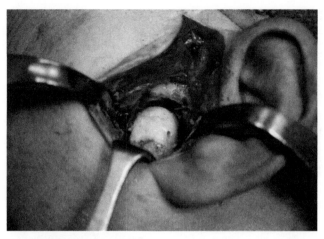

Figure 7.11 Costochondral graft well seated in the glenoid fossa.

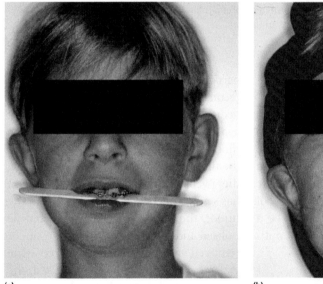

(a)

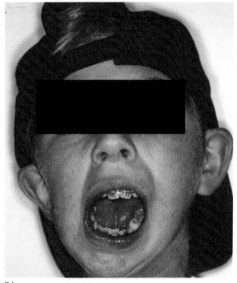

(b)

Figure 7.12 Patient following costochondral grafting (a) demonstrating good function and adaptation of the graft (b). Source: Quinn 1998, figure 6.4, p. 174. Reproduced with permission of Elsevier.

Saeed *et al.* reviewed their experience with costochrondral grafting for TMJ reconstruction compared to alloplastic reconstruction and found both groups had improved function and pain scores, but found the costochondral group required more revisions. Henry and Wolford compared their results with TMJ reconstruction using autogenous grafts compared to alloplastic total joints and found a significantly better result with the alloplastic joint reconstruction

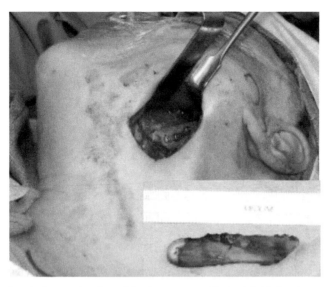

Figure 7.13 Costochondral reconstruction of the temporomandibular joint following resection of an osteochondroma. Case courtesy of Dr. Gary Warburton.

in patients with previously failed procedures. Tang *et al.* noted fewer complications in alloplastic joint reconstruction following tumor resection when compared to costochondral grafting. With the exception of reconstructing the TMJ in a previous irradiated field or use in the skeletally immature patient, the use of an alloplastic total joint appears to be a more predictable surgical option to optimize outcomes.

Vascularized (fibula) graft

Vascularized bone grafts offer the advantage of transferring large volumes of both soft tissue and bone for mandibular and temporomandibular reconstruction. These grafts are particularly ideal for patients who have received, or will receive, radiation therapy. The vascularized fibular free flap is particularly suited for temporomandibular reconstruction with its tubular shape, long pedicle, volume of bone and soft tissue available, as well as minimal donor site morbidity. Ideally, reconstruction occurs at the time of resection. When reconstructing the TMJ with a fibular graft, the surgeon has several options. If uninvolved with the tumor, the native condylar stump can be utilized and attached to the fibula in situ or removed and reattached as a free bone graft. If the condylar head is resected, the fibula may be inserted directly into the glenoid fossa. If possible, the disc is preserved. The fibula may be contoured prior to being placed into the fossa. Finally, the vascularized bone graft can be used to ensure adequate bone stock for a prosthetic device. Once the fibula is fixated, to prevent condylar sag, most surgeons advocate either suturing the pterygoid muscles to the hardware, repairing the pterygomasseteric

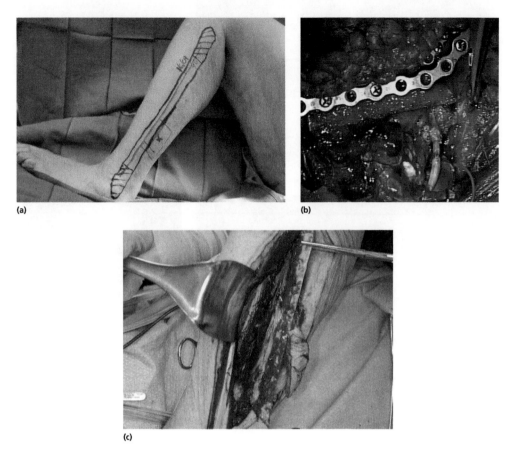

Figure 7.14 Fibular free flap used for reconstruction of the temporomandibular joint with fibula outlined (a), fibula exposed (c), and fibula inset with fixation hardware in place (b). Case courtesy of Dr. Gary Warburton.

sling or placing suspension sutures. As with all joint reconstruction, postoperative physical therapy is paramount to successful outcomes.

Distraction osteogenesis

Distraction osteogenesis offers many advantages for TMJ reconstruction. This includes the ability to reconstruct the ramus, the use of native bone, lack of donor site morbidity, single-staged resection and reconstruction, the inclusion of soft-tissue neogenesis, and no requirement for immobilization or maxillomandibular fixation. Several challenges and potential complications may occur when deploying this technique. Scarring, particularly from the pin site, can occur. Additionally, malocclusion, device failure, graft resorption, and nonunion have been reported. Obtaining correct vectors with the transport segment can be challenging, particularly with severe facial asymmetry or if a maxillary cant is present. Recent

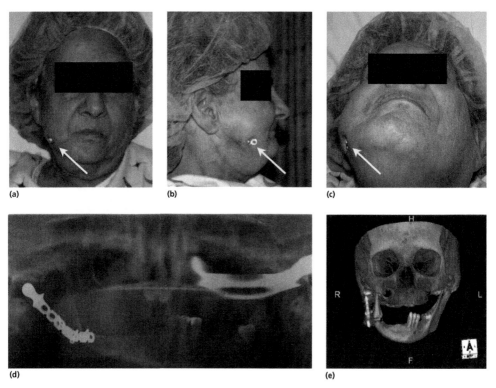

Figure 7.15 (a–c) A 68-year-old patient with a history of benign tumor resection and reconstruction with a reconstruction plate with condylar component. Recent history of recurrent infection and hardware exposure (arrow). (d) Panorex showing failed hardware. (e) 3D reconstruction demonstrating failed hardware and mandibular defect. Case courtesy of Dr. Gary Warburton.

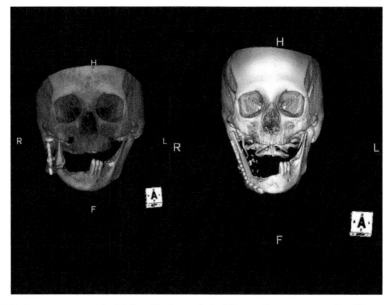

Figure 7.16 Patient reconstructed with free fibular graft. Left image shows preoperative 3D reconstruction with failed reconstruction plate and condylar component. Right image shows postoperative fibula in place with restitution of the normal mandibular contour. Case courtesy of Dr. Gary Warburton.

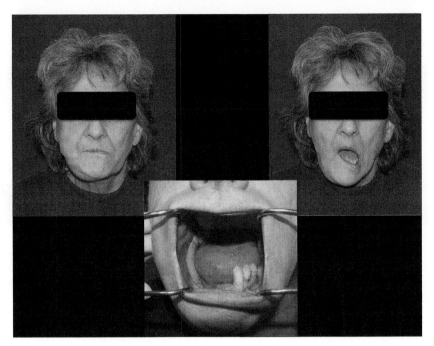

Figure 7.17 Patient following fibular reconstruction with excellent functional status and skeletal symmetry. Case courtesy of Dr. Gary Warburton.

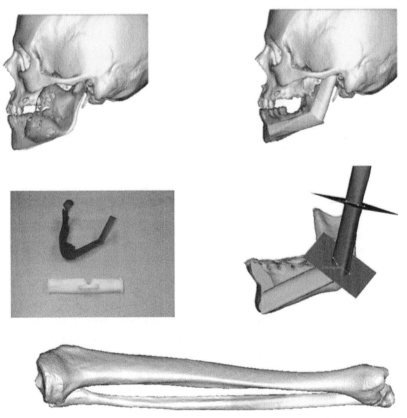

Figure 7.18 Virtual surgical planning utilized for resection and reconstruction of the temporomandibular joint with a fibula. Virtual planning can assure correct angulation and position of the fibula into the glenoid fossa. Fabricated cutting guides aid to ensure surgical planning is executed intraoperatively. Case courtesy of Dr. Gary Warburton.

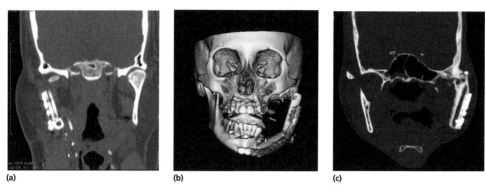

(a) (b) (c)

Figure 7.19 Complications of fibula reconstruction in the temporomandibular joint. (a) Resorption of graft to the level of the reconstruction plate with resultant asymmetry and pain. (b) 3D reconstruction of malpositioned fibula graft, with lateral displacement and articulation in the glenoid fossa. (c) Ankylosis of the graft to the skull base. (b, c) Images courtesy of Dr. Gary Warburton.

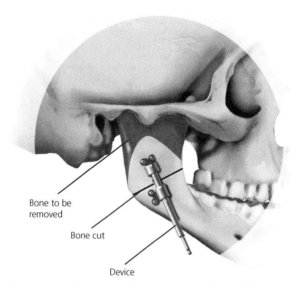

Bone to be removed

Bone cut

Device

Figure 7.20 Diagram showing area of necessary bone resection (red) and placement of distractor device. Correct angulation and device positioning are essential for good outcomes in temporomandibular joint reconstruction.

advances in multidirectional distractors and computer-aided CT planning have aided in optimizing surgical outcomes, but soft-tissue scarring and muscle contracture can still complicate the outcome. The need to line the glenoid fossa with soft tissue or disc remnant is controversial, as some authors report the formation of cartilage along the transport segment or the formation of a pseudo-disk, negating the need for fossa reconstruction. A neo-condyle should be incorporated into the

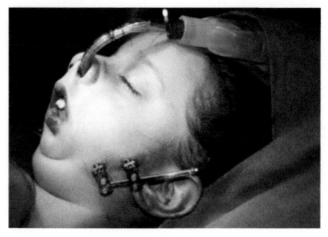

Figure 7.21 Patient with distraction device in place.

osteotomy design of the transport segment. As with all distraction osteogenesis, a latency, distraction, and consolidation period are employed. Many surgeons advocate for "overdistraction" in order to compensate for graft resorption.

Further reading

Bartlett SP. *et al.* (2006) Severe proliferative congenital temporomandibular joint ankylosis: a proposed treatment protocol utilizing distraction osteogenesis. *J Craniofac Surg,* 17:605–610.

El-Sheikh MM, Medra AM. (1997) Management of unilateral temporomandibular ankylosis associated with facial asymmetry. *J Craniomaxillofac Surg,* 25:109–115.

Gonzalez-Garcia R. *et al.* (2008) Vascularized fibular flap for reconstruction of the condyle after mandibular ablation. *J Oral Maxillofac Surg,* 66:1133–1137.

Guyot L. *et al.* (2004) Long-term radiologic findings following reconstruction of the condyle with fibular free flaps. *J Craniomaxillofac Surg,* 32:98–102.

Guyuron BC, Lasa CJ. (1992) Unpredictable growth pattern of costochondral graft. *Plast Reconstr Surg,* 90: 880–886.

Henry CH, Wolford LM. (1993) Treatment outcomes for temporomandibular joint reconstruction after failed proplast-teflon implant failed. *J Oral Maxillofac Surg,* 51:352.

Kaban LB. *et al.* 2009 A protocol for management of temporomandibular joint ankylosis in children. *J Oral Maxillofac Surg,* 67:1966–1978.

Khadka A, Hu J. (2012) Autogenous grafts for condylar reconstruction in treatment of TMJ ankylosis: current concepts and considerations for the future. *Int J Oral Maxillofac Surg,* 41:94–102.

Potter JK, Dierks EJ. (2008) Vascularized options for reconstruction of the mandibular condyle. *Semin Plast Surg,* 22:156–160.

Saeed NR. *et al.* (2002) Reconstruction of the temporomandibular joint autogenous compared with alloplastic. *Br J Oral Maxillofac Surg,* 40:296–299.

Schwartz HC, Relle RJ. (2008) Distraction osteogenesis for temporomandibular joint reconstruction. *J Oral Maxillofac Surg,* 667: 718–723.

Tang W. *et al.* (2009) Condylar replacement after tumor resection: comparison of individual prefabricated titanium implants and costochondral grafts. *Oral Surg Oral Med Oral Pathol Oral Radiol Endod,* 108: 147–152.

Vega LG. *et al.* (2013) Reconstruction of acquired temporomandibular joint defects. *Oral Maxillofac Clin North Am,* 25:251–269.

Yu H. *et al.* (2009) Gap arthroplasty combined with distraction osteogenesis in the treatment of unilateral ankylosis of the temporomandibular joint and micrognathia. *Br J Oral Maxillofac Surg,* 47:200–204.

CHAPTER 8

Stock alloplastic reconstruction of the temporomandibular joint

Reconstruction of the temporomandibular joint can be a vexing problem. Currently the accepted indications for joint reconstruction are as follows:

- Severe degenerative joint disease (osteoarthritis, rheumatoid arthritis, traumatic arthritis, etc.)
- Recurrent ankylosis
- Irreparable condyle fracture
- Revision procedures (failed alloplastic or autogenous reconstruction)
- Avascular necrosis
- Neoplasia requiring extensive resection
- Congenital disorders (e.g., hemifacial-microsomia, Treacher-Collins syndrome)

A predictably successful autogenous joint replacement would obviously be the procedure of choice rather than an alloplastic implant. An autogenous joint replacement obviates the need for the inevitable revision surgeries indicated for currently available alloplastic replacements. Autogenous joint replacement particularly costochondral grafts, are always preferred for growing patients. The chief disadvantages associated with autogenous grafts are donor-site morbidity and the variability of biologic responses (e.g., resorption, ankylosis, and excessive growth). Alloplastic joint reconstruction currently offers several advantages over autogenous replacement. These include lack of donor morbidity, reduced intra-operative surgical time, immediate functioning, the ability to correct malocclusion (with bilateral replacement) and most importantly improved predictability.

Unacceptable failure rates in previous iterations of alloplastic TMJ implant systems provided valuable input for the development of newer FDA-approved implants. Appreciation of biomechanical and orthopedic principals, along with appropriate clinical trials, has helped in the development of safe and effective devices. It is important to recognize that these devices still have limitations. This includes a finite life expectancy, limited translation, the development of wear debris, and potential for infection. As fewer patients are requiring revision arthroplasty from previous failed devices, it can be expected that more primary joint reconstruction will be performed for conditions such as severe inflammatory arthritides, trauma, and ankylosis. A stock prosthetic device has the advantage of immediate availability, single stage surgery, does not require recapitulation

---

Atlas of Temporomandibular Joint Surgery, Second Edition. Edited by Peter D. Quinn and Eric J. Granquist.
© 2015 John Wiley & Sons, Inc. Published 2015 by John Wiley & Sons, Inc.
Companion Website: www.wiley.com/go/quinn/atlasTMJsurgery

Table 8.1 Early alloplastic TMJ prostheses.

Author	Year	Material Used	Prosthesis Type
Carnochan	1840	Wood	Interpositional
Ridson	1933	Gold foil	Interpositional
Eggers	1946	Tantalum foil	Interpositional
Goodsell	1947	Tantalum foil	Interpositional
Robinson	1960	Stainless steel	Fossa
Christensen	1963–71	Chrome–cobalt	Fossa
Morgan	1971	Chrome–cobalt	Condyle
Homsy	1972	Chrome–cobalt with Proplast head	Condyle
Morgan	1973	Vitallium mesh with Acrylic head	Condyle

from a stereolithic model, and lower cost. Contraindications to alloplastic joint placement include the presence of active infection, skeletal immaturity, and severe or compromised bone deformity. Patients with severe bone anatomic discrepancies may be candidates for patient-matched custom implants.

The history of alloplastic TMJ reconstruction has been characterized by failures secondary to inappropriate design, poor clinical trial design, and failure to incorporate lesions learned from the orthopedic literature. It is important to evaluate orthopedic experience because of its longer history of joint replacement, larger volume, and greater research resources. It is equally important to realize the limitation of generalizing this knowledge to the TMJ. Wear debris is the most common mechanism for long-term device failure in artificial hips. Wear rate can be affected by too large or too small clearance values between the articular cup and condylar head. Decreased clearance can increase friction while poor matching (increased clearance) can result in lipping or dislocation and can cause material fatigue. Not only is wear rate important, but so is wear particle size and location. Many models of wear show an exponential increase in wear rates once particles begin to interact with the contact surface. This is known as the third-body wear phenomenon. Particle size can influence the biologic response. Particles in the range 0.2–7 μ can become phagocytized by macrophages resulting in proinflammatory cytokine release, osteolytic bone resorption, and potential device failure. Van Loon *et al.* evaluated wear testing of ultra-high-molecular-weight polyethylene (UHMWPE) against a metal ball in a TMJ joint system. They found the wear rate to be in an acceptable range of 0.47 mm^3/10^6 cycles confirming these to be appropriate materials for a TMJ prosthetic joint. More importantly, Westermark evaluated the histologic findings in soft tissue samples obtained around TMJ prosthetic joints of both of the available systems (Biomet and TMJ Concepts). They noted dense fibrous connective tissue without the evidence of

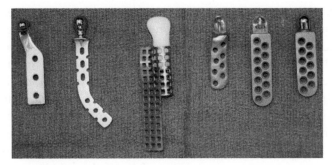

Figure 8.1 Alloplastic condylar prostheses. Left to right: Kent-Vitek, Synthes, Delrin-Timesh, Type-I Christensen, Type-II Christensen, Type-III Christensen.

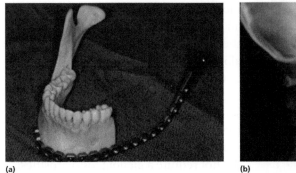

(a)

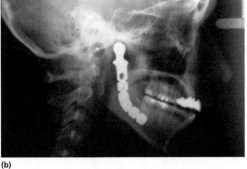

(b)

Figure 8.2 (a) Model of resected mandible with adapted reconstruction plate and attached condylar head component. (b) Postoperative image showing reconstruction plate with condylar head.

inflammation or foreign body reaction. Of interest, some samples showed evidence of synovial-like tissue. This is in contrast to reports of foreign-body reactions and metallosis seen in metal-on-metal joint systems in the TMJ. Further research is needed to better understand the finite life expectancy of the current joint systems in use.

Initially, alloplastic materials were used almost exclusively for recurrent ankylosis. Eggers used tantalum foil in 1946 as an inter-positional implant. In 1960, Robinson used a stainless-steel fossa prosthesis and Christensen used an array of cast Vitallium fossae that were secured to the zygomatic arch.

Although several attempts were made to create a condylar prosthesis, the most commonly used one was the AO–ASIF prosthesis marketed by Synthes. This type of prosthesis was essentially an extended reconstruction plate with a rounded condylar head. It was used without a matching glenoid fossa implant, as a temporary replacement. Surgeons did use the prosthesis in combination with a Vitek-Kent (VK) fossa. The VK fossa was developed in concert with the VK condylar prosthesis. Because both these components used Proplast (polytetrafluoroethylene) as a laminant, they were prone to foreign-body reaction from polymeric

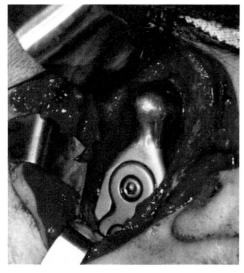

Figure 8.3 Example of two-piece reconstruction plate with condylar head.

debris. Although several authors reported long-term successes with the VK system, it is no longer manufactured, largely because of problems associated with polytetrafluoroethylene. When removing this implant system, surgeons should be aware that the ramal prosthesis was secured with a bolt-and-nut fixation, with the nuts being placed on the medial surface of the inferior ramus. Surgeons must be especially careful to remove all the Proplast both from the superior surface of the fossa implant and from the medial surface of the condylar strut. In addition, care must be taken to remove the nut fixating the condylar component along the medial surface of the mandible of the condylar strut.

In the late 1980s, Boyne reported a series of joint replacements using a Delrin (polyoxymethylene) head secured to a titanium mesh plate. Although this method did not require a glenoid fossa prosthesis, some experts were concerned about Delrin-induced excessive heterotopic bone formation, leading to ankylosis

The Christensen stock prosthesis utilizes a cobalt–chromium alloy fossa

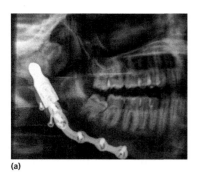

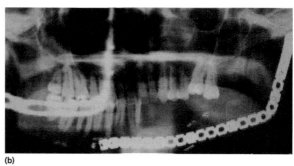

(a)   (b)

Figure 8.4 (a and b) Example of reconstruction plates with condylar component fixed. The condylar component articulates against the natural fossa, typically against an intact disk. The condylar component is indicated for temporary use and not as a definitive joint reconstruction. Images courtesy of Dr. Anders Westermark.

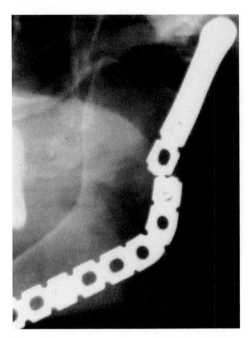

Figure 8.5 Fracture reconstruction plate with condylar head component. Images courtesy of Dr. Anders Westermark.

implant. These fossa components are 0.5 mm thick and available in approximately 40 sizes for the right and left sides. The implants are secured to the eminence and lateral border of the zygomatic arch with 2.0-mm screws. The original matching condylar prosthesis was a cobalt–chromium alloy with a methyl-methacrylate head. The type I-Christensen condylar was associated with fracture of the condylar component; however, since the advent of the type II-Christensen condylar prosthesis, which has an increased thickness and offset screw holes to avoid horizontal placement of the screws, the incidence has lessened. Currently, TMJ Medical manufactures the condylar prosthesis and TMJ Fossa-Eminence system in an all-metallic

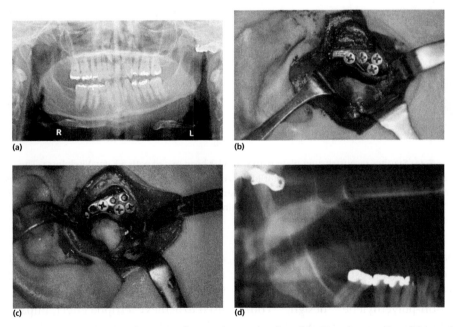

Figure 8.6 (a) Panorex showing Christensen fossa against a natural condyle. Note degeneration of the condyle. (b) Intraoperative image showing condyle against a Christensen fossa with extensive degeneration. (c) Initial hemiarthroplasty with Christensen fossa in place. (d) Postoperative image of patient with hemiarthroplasty.

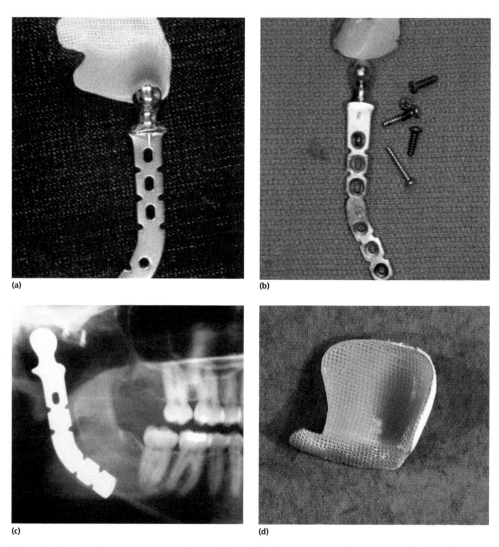

(a)

(b)

(c)

(d)

Figure 8.7 (a) Synthes reconstruction plate with condylar head mated with a Kent-Vitek fossa. The round shape of the condylar head allowed for improved mating with the fossa prosthesis. (b) Prosthesis after removal. (c) Panorex showing a Synthes reconstruction with a condylar head articulating against a Kent-Vitek fossa. (d) Photo of Kent-Vitek fossa showing the articulating surface.

(cobalt-chromium-molybdenum alloy), metal-on-metal prosthesis.

The Biomet stock prosthesis is a metal-on-polyethylene design, composed of a high-molecular-weight polyethylene fossa and a cobalt–chromium alloy condylar component. The articular eminence surface is flattened before fitting begins. A Lucite template is used to achieve a tripod effect, imparting stability to the fossa prosthesis. The fossa should parallel Frankfort horizontal or

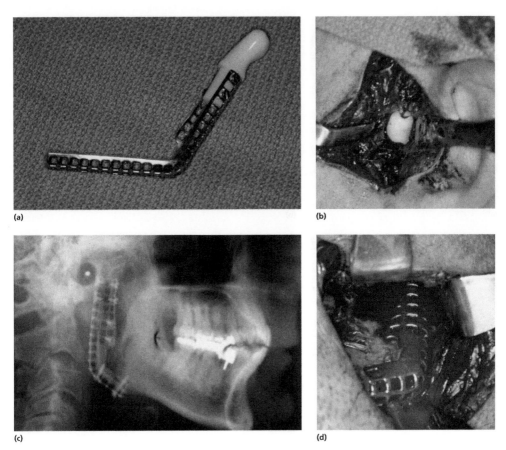

(a)

(b)

(c)

(d)

Figure 8.8 (a) Delrin-Timesh condylar prosthesis. Titanium mesh is secured directly to the posterior–inferior border of the mandible with self-tapping screws. A step osteotomy is required at the posterior–superior ramal border to allow seating of the condylar component. (b) Delrin prosthetic condyle seated in the glenoid fossa. (c) Lateral skull film showing Delrin-titanium prosthesis in place. (d) Posterior mandibular incision with a view of the posterior ramus and angle of the mandible showing adaption of the titanium mesh to the mandible.

angled slightly inferior in relation to the anterior margin to optimize function and reduce the chance of dislocation. The fossa is secured to the zygomatic arch by four self-tapping 2.0-mm screws. Once the fossa is fitted, the patient is placed in intermaxillary fixation and the chrome–cobalt condylar prosthesis is fitted. The condylar component is available in three sizes as well as a narrow or standard footplate depending on available bone for fixation. The components are designed to optimize contact between the condyle and the fossa. The point of rotation is moved inferiorly, because of the thickness of the fossa and this has improved the maximum intra-incisal opening by approximately 15–18%. Recent retrospective review of this system found significant reductions in pain and improved jaw

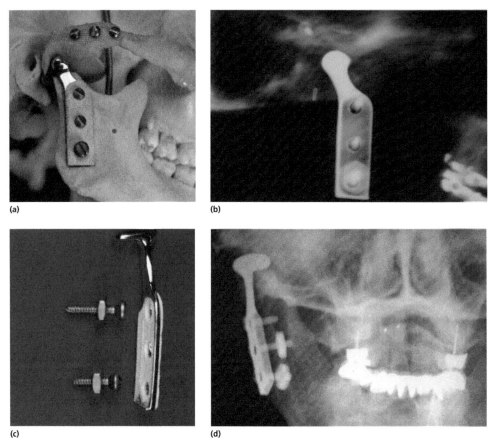

(a)　　(b)

(c)　　(d)

Figure 8.9 (a) Kent-Vitek total joint prosthesis. Note that Proplast was used for the lining of the glenoid fossa prosthesis on the fossa side and also on the surface of the condylar prosthesis itself. (b) Lateral view of the prosthesis in place. (c) Note the nut-and-bolt type of fixation. (d) Anterior–posterior view of the Kent-Vitek prosthesis showing the bolts on the medial surface of the ramus.

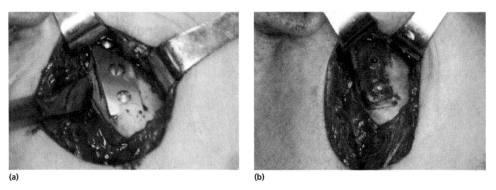

(a)　　(b)

Figure 8.10 (a) Kent-Vitek mandibular component prior to removal, note the bone overgrowth.
(b) Lateral aspect of mandibular ramus after removal of Kent-Vitek prosthesis with bone resorption.

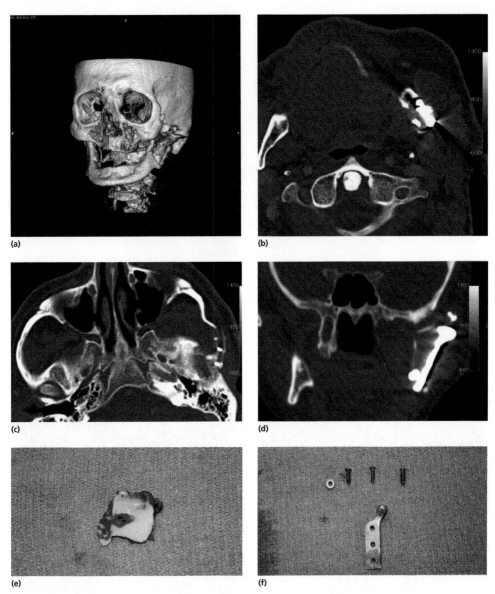

Figure 8.11 (a) CT 3D reconstruction showing extensive resorption of the left ramus secondary to a Kent-Vitek prosthesis. (b) Axial CT showing resorption around the ramus prosthesis of the Kent-Vitek prosthesis. (c) Axial CT showing resorption of zygomatic arch and screws. (d) Coronal CT showing lateral displacement of the failed prosthesis. Note nut on the medial aspect of the ramus. (e, f) Fossa, condyle, screws, and nut of Kent-Vitek prosthesis following removal.

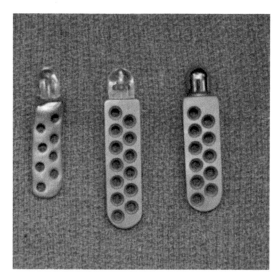

Figure 8.12 Three generation of the Chistensen prostheses, from left-to-right Christensen type 1, Christensen type II, and the all-metallic version. Note the methyl-methacrylate head of the type-I and type-II prosthesis.

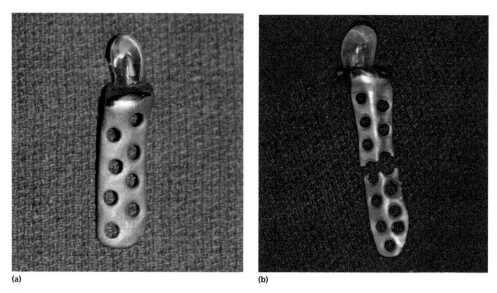

(a)   (b)

Figure 8.13 (a) Type I-Christensen condylar prosthesis. (b) Fracture of prosthesis at the point of screw holes that were not angle-offset.

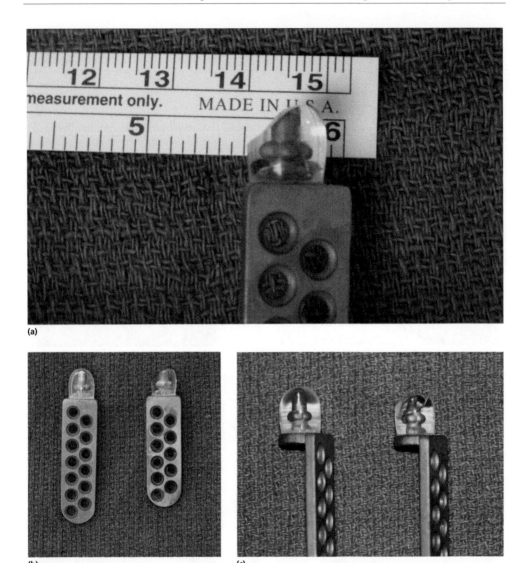

Figure 8.14 (a) Wear of methyl-methacrylate head of Christensen type-II prosthesis. Note wear to level of pin. (b) Lateral view of wear to condylar head (right) compared to a new prosthetic device (left). (c) Oblique view of wear of condylar (right) head compared to a new device (left).

function. No mechanical failures were seen and a 3.2% device removal rate was reported (e.g., infection or heterotopic bone formation).

Hemiarthroplasty or partial joint reconstruction with an alloplastic fossa-eminence replacement against a native condyle has been described in the TMJ.

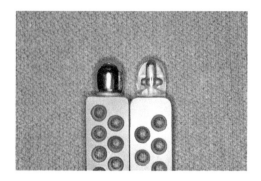

Figure 8.15 Comparison of condylar head from the all-metal version currently available and the Christensen Type-II prosthesis.

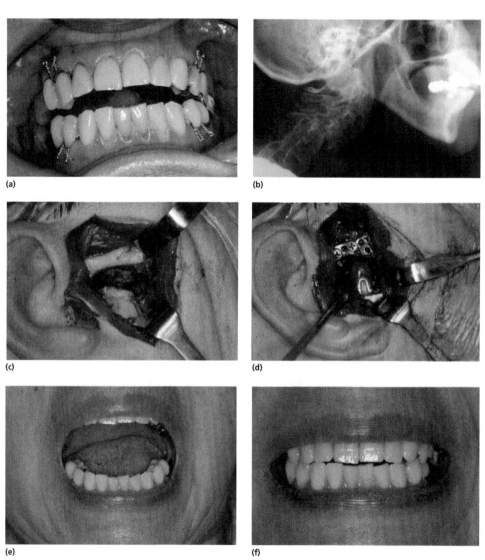

Figure 8.16 (a) Anterior open bite secondary to progressive bilateral condylar resorption in a patient with advanced rheumatoid arthritis. (b) Lateral skull film showing a "swan-neck" cervical deformity. (c) Open view of the joint after removal of the adhesions, note severe degeneration of the condylar head, cartilage, and loss of height. (d) Christensen I total joint prosthesis positioned during intermaxillary fixation. (e, f) Postoperative opening and occlusion.

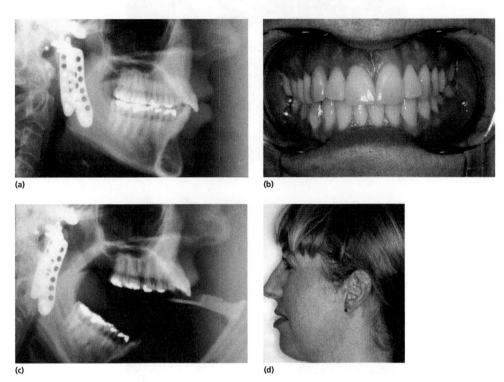

Figure 8.17 (a) Lateral cephalogram showing bilateral Christensen I total joint prostheses in closed mouth position. (b) Postoperative occlusion. (c) Lateral cephalogram showing bilateral Christensen total joints during maximal opening with the aid of a hand-held jaw exerciser. (d) Note well-concealed appearance of the endaural and retromandibular incisions. Source for (d): Quinn 1998, figure 7.29a, p. 192. Reproduced with permission of Elsevier.

Indications for use are similar to total joint replacement but have primarily been described for use in patients with osteoarthritis to prevent bone-on-bone contact and ankylosis in patients with severe degeneration. Advantages include preservation of translation and lateral movements of the joint, decreased cost, and decreased loss of native tissue. Specific disadvantages include increased resorption and wear of the native condyle and progressive occlusal changes.

A complete understanding of the biomechanics and occlusal considerations of the patient requiring total alloplastic joint reconstruction is essential. Translational and rotational movements, as well as bite force and speech function need to be taken into consideration with prosthetic joint design and surgical placement. The function of patients requiring joint replacement is often severely diminished preoperatively. This is often secondary to pain, scar formation, or ankylosis.

Careful preoperative planning and reasonable patient expectations are required for successful joint reconstruction. A maximal opening between 30 and

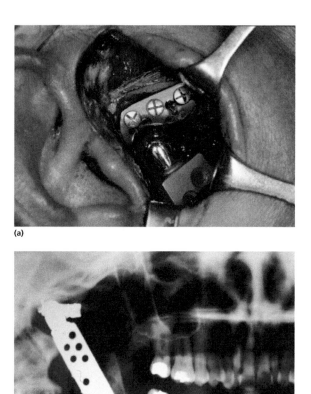

(a)

(b)

Figure 8.18 (a) Christensen all-metal condylar prosthesis articulating with a Christensen fossa. Both components are made with Vitallium. (b) A panorex film showing the all-metal Christensen prosthesis in position.

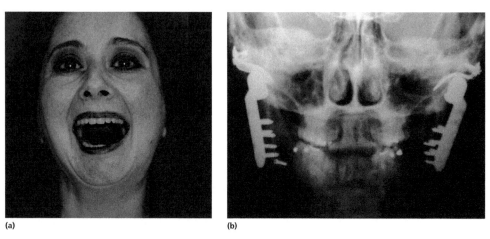

(a)   (b)

Figure 8.19 (a) Thirty-one-year-old woman who underwent bilateral total joint replacement with all-metal Christensen prostheses after several unsuccessful arthroplasties. The interincisal opening is 32 mm. (b) Anterior–posterior skull view of all-metal Christensen prostheses. Source: Quinn 1998, figure 7.45, p. 205. Reproduced with permission of Elsevier.

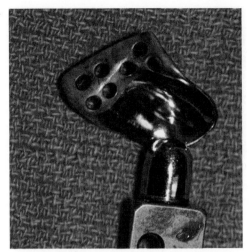

Figure 8.20 Christensen all-metal total prosthetic joint (post-removal).

35mm is a reasonable expectation for range of motion with a total joint prosthesis. Failure to achieve this range of motion intraoperatively may require coronoidectomy or muscle stripping. Patient with prolonged decreased range of motion often have muscle and soft tissue contracture and scarring. The patient should be aware that unilateral replacement causes deviation to the side of the prosthesis on terminal opening. Pain reduction for patients who have undergone multiple operations is often difficult to achieve; a direct correlation exists between the number of previous surgical procedures and the likelihood that presurgical

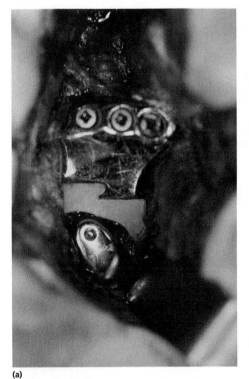

(a)

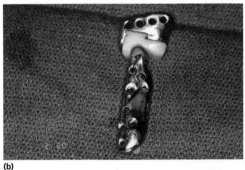

(b)

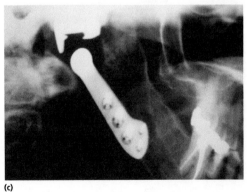

(c)

Figure 8.21 (a) Intraoperative image showing the Endotec prosthesis in place. This prosthesis system was a "plastic on metal" design with a removable fossa component (b). (c) Panorex showing the Endotec prosthesis in place. The condylar component is secured with locking screws.

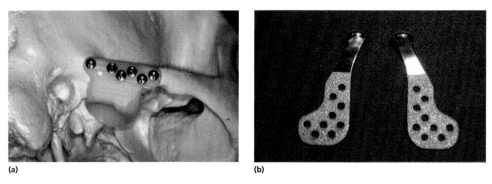

(a)   (b)

Figure 8.22 (a) Model showing correct position of Biomet fossa prosthesis. (b) Biomet Mandibular prosthesis, which is an alloy of chromium, cobalt, and molybdenum with a titanium-coated medial surface.

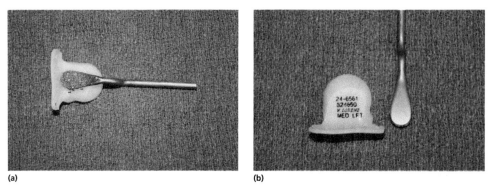

(a)   (b)

Figure 8.23 (a and b) Rasp overlying fossa; note that the length of rasp matches width of the glenoid surface of the fossa. The rasp is used to reduce and flatten the articular eminence, and this allows for tripod stability of the fossa component.

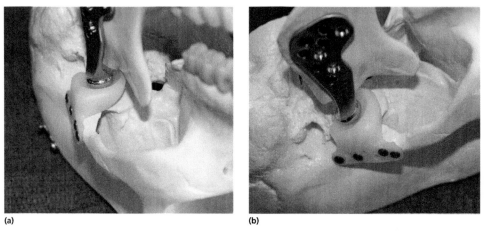

(a)   (b)

Figure 8.24 (a and b) Biomet total joint system on model skull. Note matching of the condylar component and fossa.

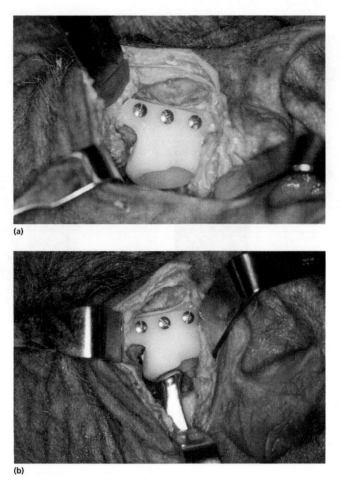

(a)

(b)

Figure 8.25 (a) Biomet fossa in place on a cadaver. (b) Demonstration of "pseudo-translation" which occurs with unilateral placement from the contralateral lateral pterygoid muscle.

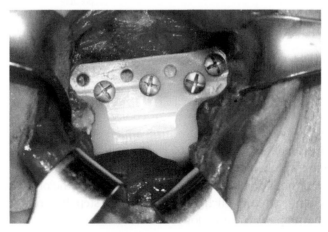

Figure 8.26 Biomet fossa component in place. Note placement of a minimum of four screws, with three additional holes present for additional screws if necessary for added stability. If necessary, large size fossas are available with a longer flange for more screw hole options, if the zygomatic arch is compromised.

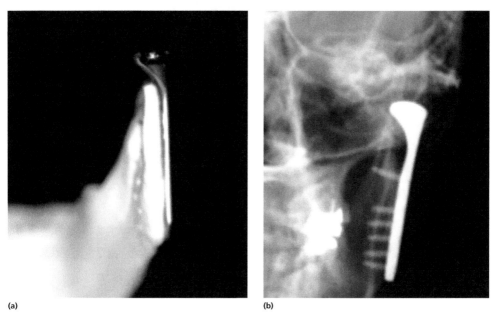

(a)   (b)

Figure 8.27 (a) Model showing correct place of the condylar component of the Biomet total joint system. Note the level of the osteotomy to accommodate the "swan-neck" shape of the prosthesis. (b) Posterior–anterior skull film with prosthesis in place.

Table 8.2 Comparison of stock and custom alloplastic devices.

	Stock prosthesis	Custom prosthesis
Advantages	• Immediately available • Flexibility • Lower cost	• Address anatomic defects • Patient-matched • Excessive anteroinferior movements possible
Disadvantages	• Limited anteroinferior movements • Surgeon modification required	• Higher cost • Limited flexibility (must replicate model surgery)

symptoms will be reduced. A preoperative antibiotic should be given 1 hour prior to incision to ensure adequate tissue levels. At our institution, patients are given cefazolin and metronidazole, unless a penicillin allergy is present, in which case clindamycin is the prophylactic antibiotic of choice. All components are soaked in an antibiotic solution prior to implantation. Attention to sterile technique, especially when alternating between the surgical site and the oral cavity, is the most important step in preventing prosthetic infection.

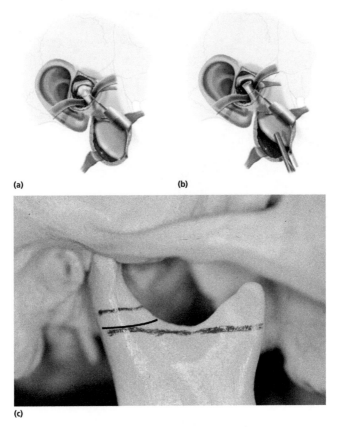

(a)

(b)

(c)

Figure 8.28 Two-step osteotomy. (a) Initial condylectomy with use of Dunn-Dautrey retractors to protect deeper structures. (b) Superior repositioning of the ramus to allow for improved access to the second-stage osteotomy and avoidance of the internal maxillary artery. (c) The location of two-step osteotomies, note curvilinear shape of black line if coronoidectomy is not required.

A two-step osteotomy is recommended to minimize risk to the internal maxillary artery and ensure adequate bone removal for the fossa component. With the TMJ fully exposed, two Dunn-Dautrey retractors and a condylar neck retractor are placed deep to the condylar neck to aid in visualization and protect deeper structures. A 1-mm fissure bur is used to perform the condylectomy. An osteotomy is performed by first starting at the midpoint of the condylar neck, sparing the medial cortex. The cut is then extended both anteriorly and posteriorly. A T-bar osteotome is then used to complete the condylectomy. The condyle is then grasped with a bone holding forcep and the lateral ptyregoid is then carefully dissected free. At this point, significant bleeding may occur and the surgeon should be ready to control any hemorrhage with the aid of hemostatic agents. Once the condyle is removed, this creates space and allows

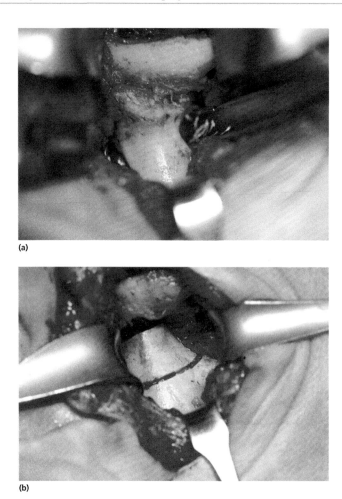

(a)

(b)

Figure 8.29 (a) Intraoperative image showing severe degeneration of the temporomandibular condyle with Dunn-Dautrey retractors in place showing excellent access prior to initial osteotomy. (b) Initial condylectomy complete, the remaining stump is superiorly positioned to allow for the second osteotomy. Superiorly repositioning the condylar stump allows for the second osteotomy to occur at a safe distance from the maxillary artery.

the surgeon to superiorly reposition the ramus. This maneuver allows easier access to the second step of the osteotomy and places this bone cut away from the internal maxillary artery. After the fossa prosthesis is placed, the patient must be placed in stable intermaxillary fixation when the condylar prosthesis is being placed. The prosthesis should be secured with two screws initially, and then the mandible should be manipulated through a range of motion to ensure that centric occlusion can be achieved and the prosthesis does not subluxate or dislocate. Ideal screw placement and position is important when planning and placing the prosthetic implants. Factors such as bone availability, bone quality, and inferior alveolar nerve position need to be taken into account when placing fixation. Hsu *et al.* studied the effect of screw number and position on prosthesis stress and stability using a three-dimensional finite model. They evaluated eight different screw configurations and found a nonlinear reduction in micromotion with each additional screw. They noted a small increase in stability when increasing from three to five screws compared to the increase from two to three screws. They also noted a more stable configuration with staggered screw placement compared to screws placed in a linear fashion. They concluded that increasing the number of screws beyond three only slightly enhances stability, and screw position is more important than quantity. Current recommendations are for the placement of a minimum of four screws in the condylar component. In addition to number and position, bone quality is another factor to consider when placing the prosthetic. In another study by Hsu *et al.*, the effect of bone quality and prosthetic stability was examined using the same model as described earlier. In this study, the micromotion and stability of the prosthetic were evaluated as the bone quality increased from type IV to type I bone. They concluded that increasing the quality of bone increased stability, but this has only a minor effect. They further concluded that surgeons placing prosthetic devices in osteoporotic patients should consider using additional screws for stabilization.

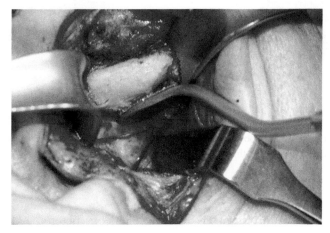

Figure 8.30 Diamond rasp used to reduce and flatten the articular eminence. Note the rasp is parallel to Frankfort horizontal to ensure correct positioning of the fossa.

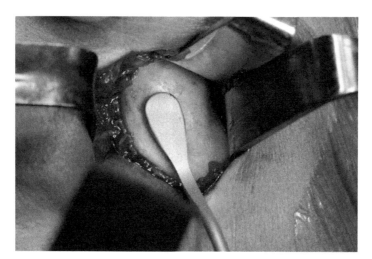

Figure 8.31 A diamond used on lateral surface of the mandible to ensure stable seating and positioning of the condylar component.

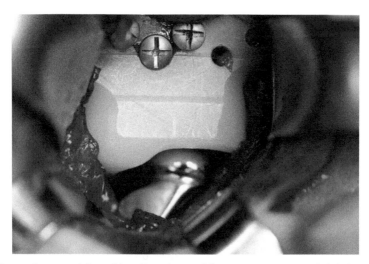

Figure 8.32 Correct fossa-condyle position. Note the condylar component is seated slightly posterior in the fossa and in the midpoint along the medial-lateral plane.

Complications that are specific to alloplastic joints include the following: prosthesis displacement or fracture, foreign-body reaction to polymeric or metallic debris, heterotopic bone formation (which causes ankylosis of the prosthesis), and damage to the inferior alveolar nerve by screw placement. The facial nerve can

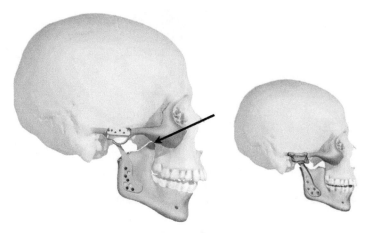

Figure 8.33 Diagram (left) shows portion of coronoid removed (arrow) during a coronoidectomy. This is necessary if maximal opening remains less than 30 mm after the condylectomy is complete and aids in freeing soft tissue restriction on mandibular motion. Diagram (right) showing coronoid removed with total joint prosthesis in place.

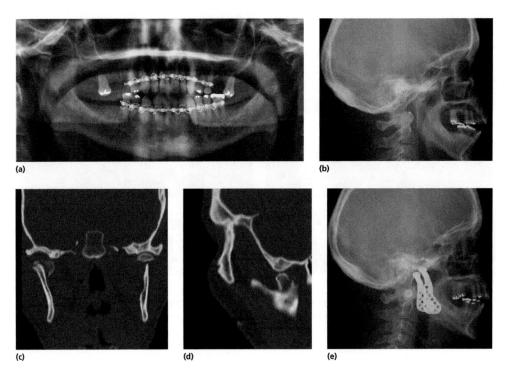

Figure 8.34 Immediate placement of total joint replacement of the TMJ in a trauma patient. (a) Note bilateral condylar head fractures. (b) Lateral cephalogram showing anterior open bite and collapse of the vertical dimension of occlusion (VDO). (c) Coronal CT showing bilateral condylar fractures. (d) Sagittal CT showing condylar head fracture causing mechanical obstruction. (e) Lateral cephalogram showing bilateral total joint replacement of the TMJ and reestablishment of VDO. Images courtesy of Dr. Sotirios Diamantis.

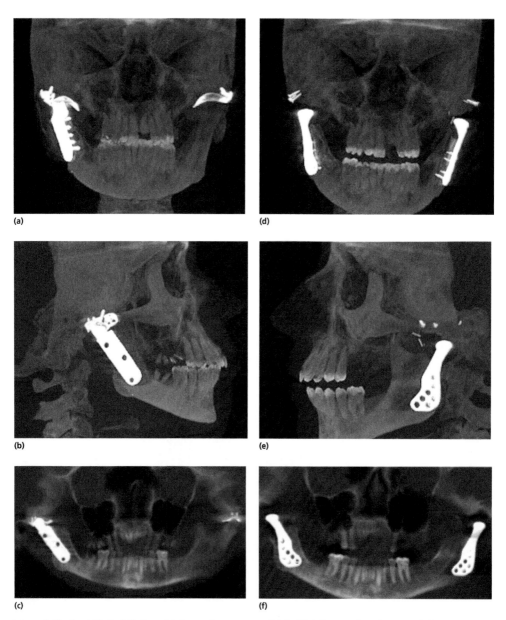

Figure 8.35 (a–c) Right failed total joint replacement and failed left hemiarthroplasty with fossa component. (d–f) Reconstruction using stock total alloplastic joint reconstruction.

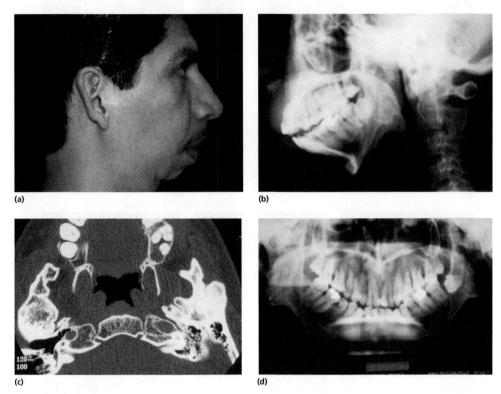

Figure 8.36 (a) Patient with bilateral ankylosis of the temporomandibular joint and resultant retrognathia. (b) Lateral cephalogram of patient, note the prominent antegonial notching and counter-clockwise rotation of the occlusal plane. (c) Axial CT of patient with bilateral ankylosis showing the medial extent of the ankylosis. (d) Panorex with complete loss of joint space and coronoid notch bilaterally. Also note the prominent antegonial notching present when ankylosis occurs in a developing patient.

be damaged during placement of the prosthesis, but this risk is inherent in all joint procedures. Complications and their management are covered in Chapter 10.

In the skeletally mature patients, a stock alloplastic total joint is a predictable, efficient, and cost effective means for joint reconstruction. Although continued research is necessary in biomaterials, pain management, and basic mechanisms of temporomandibular joint disorders, alloplastic reconstruction with an FDA-approved stock prosthesis has proven to be a safe and effective procedure for end-stage TMJ disease.

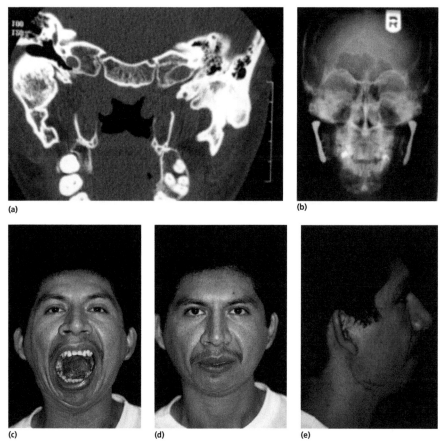

Figure 8.37 (a) Coronal CT of patient from Figure 8.35 showing bilateral temporomandibular joint ankylosis. The medial-lateral and inferior extent of the bony mass can be fully appreciated from this view. It is also important to evaluate the relation of the bony fusion to the skull base in order to minimize complications during resection. (b) Postoperative PA skull film with bilateral stock total joints in place. (c–e) Postoperative photographs of patient following joint reconstruction. Note maximal opening (c) and anterior repositioning of the mandible to improve projection (e).

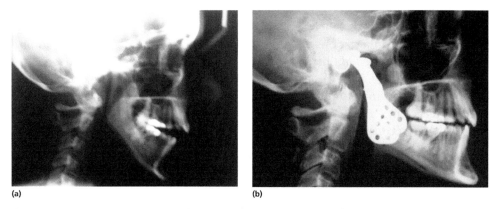

Figure 8.38 (a) Preoperative lateral cephalogram of a patient with loss of vertical dimension of occlusion and resultant anterior open bite secondary to severe degenerative temporomandibular joint disease. (b) Patient following stock total alloplastic joint reconstruction with restoration of class I occlusion.

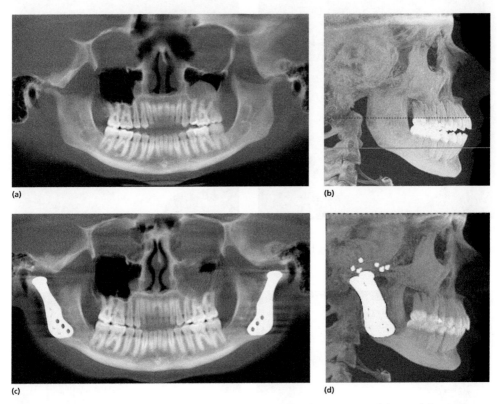

Figure 8.39 (a) Patient with psoriatic arthritis resulting in severe degeneration of the condyles and loss of vertical dimension with progressive anterior open bite. (b) Lateral 3D view showing anterior open bite and loss of normal condylar anatomy. (c) Postoperative panorex with bilateral stock alloplastic joint in place and restoration of class 1 occlusion. (d) Lateral 3D image showing prosthesis in place and appropriate mandibular projection.

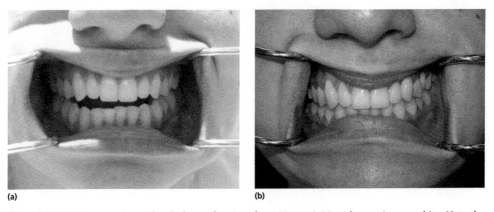

Figure 8.40 (a) Preoperative occlusal photo of patient from Figure 3.38 with anterior open bite. Note the wear pattern evident of the anterior incisors, evidence of an acquired open bite. (b) Postoperative occlusal image showing restoration of class 1 occlusion.

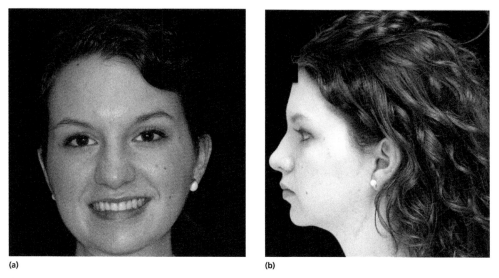

Figure 8.41 (a and b) Patient following bilateral total joint replacement. Note well-healed appearance of incisions.

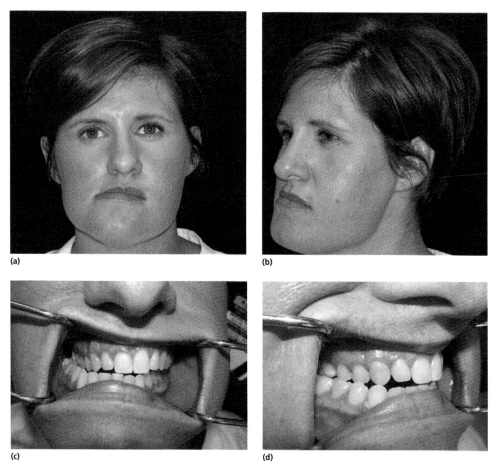

Figure 8.42 (a and b) Patient with osteochondroma of the left temporomandibular joint. Note the facial asymmetry evident in the lower third of the face. Pathology of the temporomandibular joint which occurs after facial growth is complete will not affect midface structures. (c and d) Occlusal images showing deviation of the mandible and normal maxilla without cant or dental compensation.

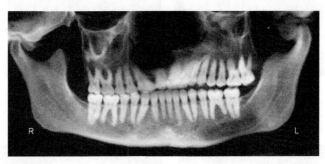

Figure 8.43 Panorex of patient in Figure 8.41. Note large condylar mass in the left temporomandibular joint (osteochondroma).

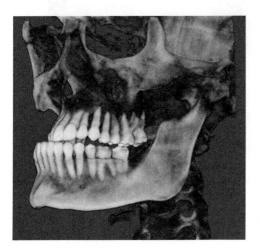

Figure 8.44 3D reconstruction showing condylar mass with deviation of the condylar from the "mass effect" in the temporomandibular joint.

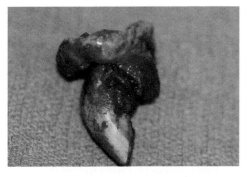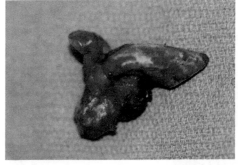

Figure 8.45 Resected osteochondroma from Figures 8.41 to 8.43 with margin of normal condylar neck.

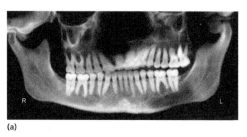
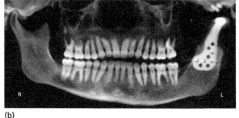

(a)   (b)

Figure 8.46 (a) Preoperative panorex and (b) postoperative panorex showing resection of osteochondroma and immediate reconstruction with a stock alloplastic total joint.

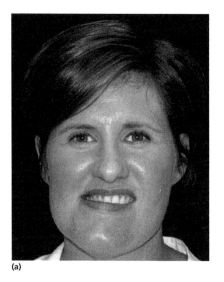
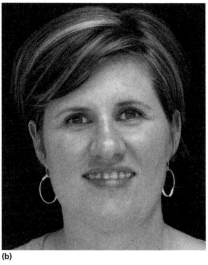

(a)   (b)

Figure 8.47 (a) Preoperative and (b) postoperative view of patient. Note facial symmetry restored following resection and immediate reconstruction.

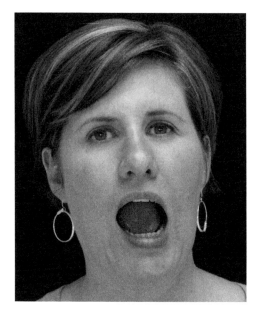

Figure 8.48 Maximal opening of patient with left total joint replacement. Patient with good function, note slight deviation to side of the prosthesis on opening.

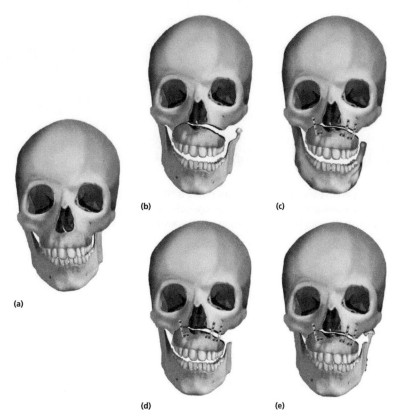

Figure 8.49 Protocol for single-staged reconstruction and restoration of facial asymmetry secondary to temporomandibular joint degeneration. (a) Skeletal asymmetry secondary to left TMJ degeneration. (b) Lefort osteotomy and repositioning based on native position of the mandible. (c) Fixation of maxilla in new position. (d) Condylectomy of diseased left temporomandibular joint and repositioning of mandible into new position set to repositioned maxilla. (e) Reconstruction of the left temporomandibular joint with stock alloplastic joint. A genioplasty may also be performed at this time if indicated.

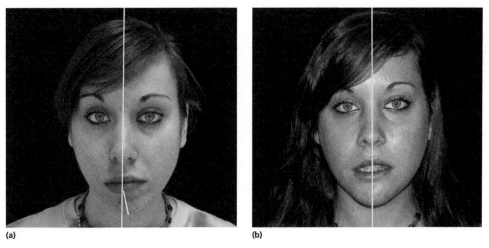

Figure 8.50 (a) Patient with psoriatic arthritis since childhood. Note facial asymmetry. (b) Patient following stock total alloplastic joint reconstruction and genioplasty with restitution of facial symmetry.

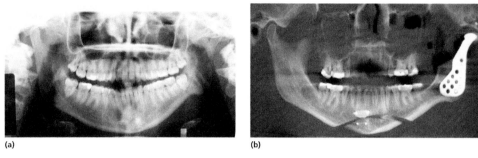

(a)   (b)

Figure 8.51 (a) Preoperative image of patient from Figure 8.50. Note left degenerative temporomandibular joint and increased left antegonial notching. (b) Postoperative imaging following Lefort osteotomy, total joint reconstruction and genioplasty for correction of facial asymmetry and joint pain and dysfunction.

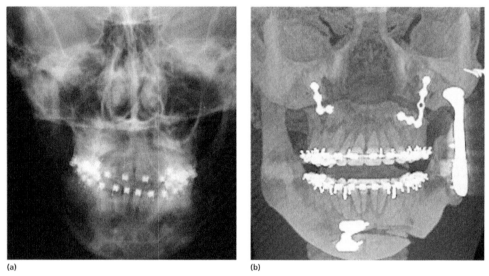

(a)   (b)

Figure 8.52 (a) Preoperative image of facial asymmetry with maxillary canting from unilateral arthritis in the temporomandibular joint in a developing patient. (b) Reconstruction including Lefort osteotomy, genioplasty, and stock alloplastic joint reconstruction in a single-staged surgery for the correction of skeletal asymmetry.

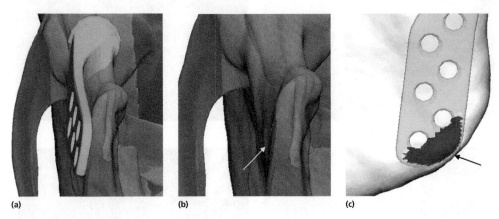

(a)   (b)   (c)

Figure 8.53 (a) Computed generated surgical plan with stock prosthesis in place. (b) Utilizing this software, allows for the evaluation of potential interference (yellow arrow). (c) Lateral view of bony interference to ideal prosthesis placement identified in the surgical planning stages. (Images courtesy of Dr. Ron Caloss)

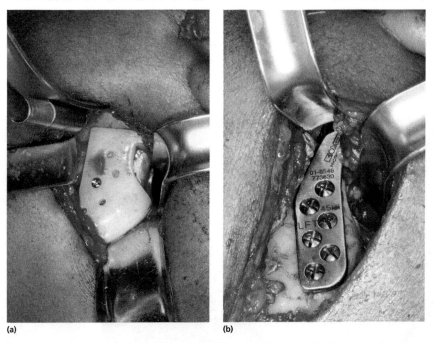

(a)   (b)

Figure 8.54 (a) Intraoperative image with cutting guide secured in place. (b) Intraoperative image with the mandibular component secured in the correct position. (Images courtesy of Dr. Ron Caloss)

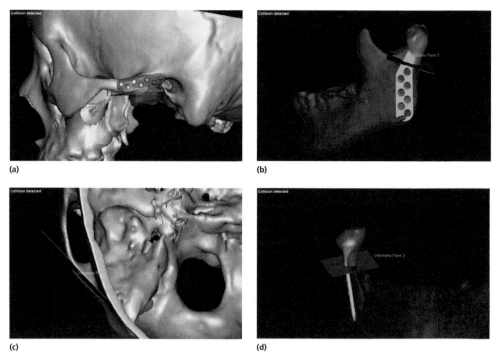

Figure 8.55 (a) Osteotomy plane for bony protuberance at the bottom of articular tubercle, and evaluation of fossa component angulation. (b) Osteotomy plane for condylar neck (sagittal view), grey part indicates condyle to be removed (c) Osteotomy plane for lateral surface of zygomatic arch. (d) Osteotomy plane for condylar neck (posterior view), the osteotomy plane has to go beneath the inner inclination of fossa prosthesis. (Images courtesy of Drs Yang, He and Bai)

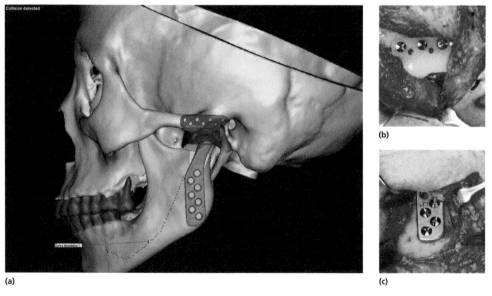

Figure 8.56 (a) 2 Ideal placement position of fossa and ramus prostheses, noted identification of inferior alveolar nerve (dotted line). (b) Implantation of the fossa prosthesis according to the location holes drilled with a prefabricated computer design cutting guide based. (c) Implantation of the ramus prosthesis according to the location holes from a cutting guide. Use of the cutting guide to set the screw holes ensure ideal position based on computer designed presurgical plan. (Images courtesy of Drs Yang, He and Bai)

Further reading

Bhatt H, Goswami T. (2008) Implant wear mechanism—basic approach. *Biomed Mater*, 3:042001.

Bradrick JP, Indresano AT. (1992) Failure rates of repetitive temporomandibular surgical procedures. *J Oral Maxillofac Surg*, 50:145.

Driemel O. *et al.* (2009) Historical development of alloplastic temporomandibular joint replacement after 1945 and state of the art. *Int J Oral Maxillofac Surg*, 38:909–920.

Giannakopoulos HE. *et al.* (2012) Biomet Microfixation temporomandibular joint replacement system: a 3-year follow-up study of patients treated during 1995 to 2005. *J Oral Maxillofac Surg*, 70:787–794.

Guarda-Nardini L. *et al.* (2008) Temporomandibular joint total replacement prosthesis: current knowledge and considerations for the future. *Int J Oral Maxillofac Surg*, 37:103–110.

Hsu J-T. *et al.* (2010) Effect of bone quality on the artificial temporomandibular joint condylar prosthesis. *Oral Surg Oral Med Oral Pathol Oral Radiol Endod*, 109:e1–e5.

Hsu J-T. *et al.* (2011) Effect of screw fixation on temporomandibular joint condylar prosthesis. *J Oral Maxillofac Surg*, 69:1320–1328.

Ingham E, Fisher J. (2000) Biological reactions to wear debris in total joint replacement. *Proc Inst Mech Eng H*, 214:21–37.

Leandro LFL. *et al.* (2013) A 10-year experience and follow-up of three hundred patients with the Biomet/Lorenz Microfixation TMJ replacement system. *Int J Oral Maxillofac Surg*, 42:1007–1013.

McGloughlin TM, Kavanagh AG. (2000) Wear of ultra-high molecular weight polyethylene (UHMWPE) in total knee prostheses: a review of key influences. *Proc Inst Mech Eng H*, 214: 349–359.

Milam SB. (1997) Failed implants and multiple operations. *Oral Surg Oral Med Oral Pathol Oral Radiol Endod*, 83:156–162.

Quinn PD. (1996) Alloplastic reconstruction of the temporomandibular joint. *Selected Read Oral Maxillofac Surg*, 7(5):1–20.

Quinn PD. (2000) Lorenz prosthesis. *Oral Maxillofac Surg Clin North Am*, 12:93–299.

Sidebottom AJ. (2008) Guidelines for the replacement of temporomandibular joints in the United Kingdom. *Br J Oral Maxillofac Surg*, 46:146–147.

Sidebottom AJ. *et al.* (2008) Foreign body response around total prosthetic metal-on-metal replacements of the temporomandibular joint in the UK. *Br J Oral Maxillofac Surg*, 46: 288–292.

Van Loon J-P. *et al.* (1995) Evaluation of temporomandibular joint prostheses: review of the literature from 1946 to 1994 and implications for future prosthesis designs. *J Oral Maxillofac Surg*, 53:984–996.

Westermark A. (2010) Total reconstruction of the temporomandibular joint. Up to 8 years follow-up of patients with Biomet total joint prostheses. *Int J Oral Maxillofac Surg*, 39:951–955.

CHAPTER 9

Custom alloplastic reconstruction of the temporomandibular joint

Introduction

Alloplastic total joint systems are available custom-designed for the patient. The use of a custom implant system is usually necessitated in cases where there is a severe craniofacial deformity present with an anatomical discrepancy, which precludes the use of a stock device. Severe deformities may be present secondary to congenital abnormalities, previous failed reconstruction, or following resection or ablative surgery. In addition, patients with compromised bone stock, often from previous radiation treatment or osteomyelitis, may benefit from the use of a custom implant system in order to optimize fixation placement to achieve primary stability. Finally, when a total joint replacement is preformed in conjunction with orthognathic surgery, particularly when large advancements or rotations of the facial skeleton are performed, a custom implant may be required, because marked angulation of a stock implant is unadvisable. Currently, three custom temporomandibular replacement systems are available (two in the United States). Two systems utilize a metal-on-polyethylene design, and one system is metal-on-metal. Though these systems are planned and designed for the patient, several disadvantages and challenges may be encountered when placing these devices. This includes larger than anticipated resection, poor bone quality in planned screw sites, osteotomy or bone contouring in the incorrect location and "over or under" bone preparation. In addition, device cost is significantly greater when compared to a stock device. Many of these disadvantages can be avoided with careful planning or with a staged operation. Proper diagnosis, planning, and implementation are paramount to any successful temporomandibular joint reconstruction. Despite this planning, the ability to alter the treatment plan when unanticipated intra-operative findings occur, may be lost with a custom device. Surgical approach, positioning, and post-operative care are the same for both stock and custom devices (see Chapter 8).

Atlas of Temporomandibular Joint Surgery, Second Edition. Edited by Peter D. Quinn and Eric J. Granquist.
© 2015 John Wiley & Sons, Inc. Published 2015 by John Wiley & Sons, Inc.
Companion Website: www.wiley.com/go/quinn/atlasTMJsurgery

Surgical planning

Prosthetic manufacturing is done using one of the two methods. The first method introduced utilizes anatomic models produced from a CT scan. These models are then used to fabricate the custom prosthesis via an initial computer-aided wax model. Utilizing this method, the reconstruction can be accomplished with a single- or two-staged approach. The two-staged reconstruction requires initial joint preparation, including tumor resection, device removal, or

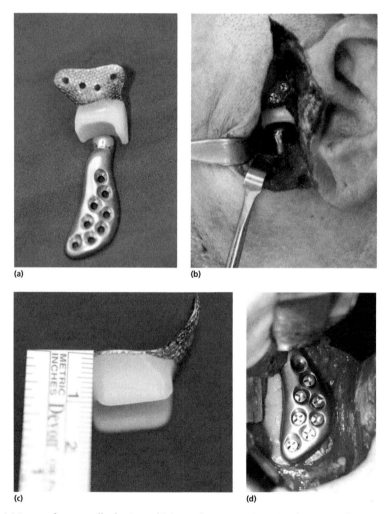

(a)

(b)

(c)

(d)

Figure 9.1 (a) Image of custom alloplastic total joint replacement prior to implantation. (b) Intraoperative imaging showing prosthesis in place and in good position. (c) Image of fossa component showing thickness of polyethylene articulating surface. It is important to perform a sufficient condylar osteotomy to ensure appropriate spacing for the fossa component. (d) Intraoperative view of condylar component in place. Exact designed placement is important to ensure appropriate position, angulation, and function (TMJ Concepts).

bony resection to occur. Once this is completed in the first operation, the patient is placed in intermaxillary fixation and a CT scan is obtained. The device is then fabricated from this scan. The advantage to this approach is that the defect and new mandibular position is set. The obvious disadvantages include a second procedure and the need for prolonged mandibular immobilization during device manufacturing. The single-stage approach requires initial site preparation and device placement in a single surgery. Planning and design are first replicated on the model surgery, with osteotomy sites and bone contouring marked. The model can be made in two pieces, allowing the mandible to be repositioned. Advantages to this technique include a single operation. Disadvantages included the need to recapitulate osteotomy and mandibular repositioning precisely as they were placed on the model. This can be accomplished by measuring anatomic points on the model, not altered by the surgery. Care must be taken while transferring these measurements intraoperatively, as soft tissue not present on the model may complicate measurement on the patient.

A second method for surgical planning and custom device design utilizes computer modeling entirely. Mandibular repositioning and osteotomy

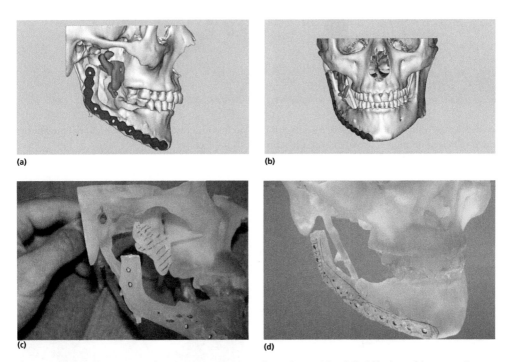

Figure 9.2 (a and b) Preoperative 3D reconstruction of a patient with a failed fibula and heterotopic bone formation. Resorption of the graft had resulted in malocclusion and pain. (c and d) Two-piece stereolithic model with occlusion set and waxed into place. Once the surgeon sets the occlusion, it is sent back to the manufacturer for the design of the prosthesis.

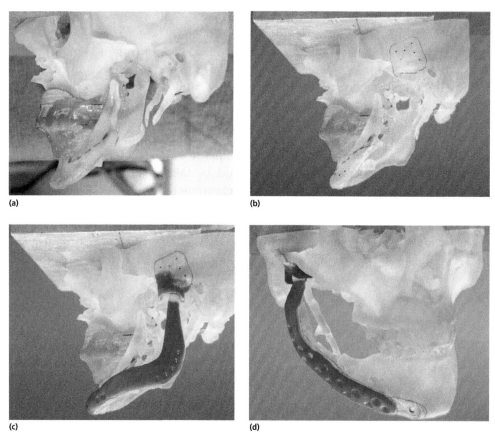

(a)   (b)   (c)   (d)

Figure 9.3 (a) Example of a two-piece model with new occlusion set. (b) Example of an initial prosthesis design indicated on model. (c and d) Wax-up of prosthesis in place.

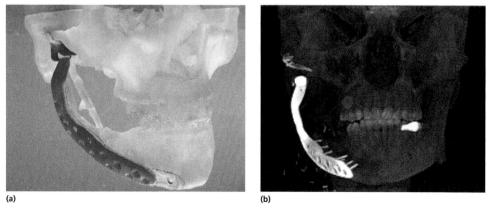

(a)   (b)

Figure 9.4 (a) Wax-up of custom prosthesis from Figure 9.3. (b) Postoperative image showing prosthesis in place and correction of malocclusion.

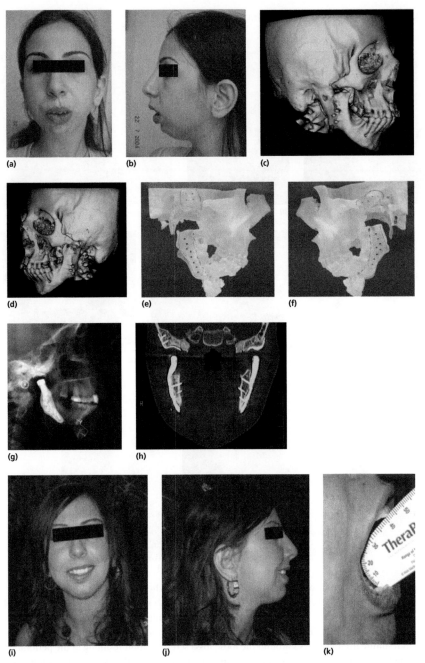

Figure 9.5 (a and b) Twenty-year-old female, bilateral TMJ ankylosis status post prepubertal bilateral mandibular condyle fractures. She has had five prior unsuccessful bilateral procedures including costochondral grafts twice, temporalis muscle flaps twice, and coronoidectomies. (c and d) 3D CT scans demonstrating bilateral complete bony TMJ ankylosis. (e and f) Stereo laser design models (ProtoMED, Westminster, CO) following stage 1 bilateral gap arthroplasties, insertion of spacer and advancement genioplasty. (g and h) Lateral cephalometric and coronal CT post stage 2 implantation of TMJ Concepts (Ventura, CA) patient-fitted prostheses. The articulating aspect of the fossa component is ultra-high-molecular weight polyethylene, and therefore it is radiolucent. (a–h) Case courtesy of Dr. Mercuri. (i–k) The patient after dental rehabilitation, 5 years post-bilateral TMJ Concepts patient-fitted replacements. Images for this case were supplied by Dr. Michael Bowler, Newcastle, New South Wales, Australia

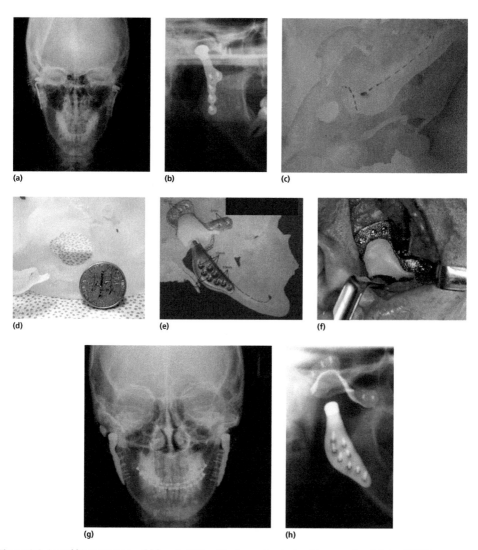

Figure 9.6 (a and b) Forty-year-old female Ehlers Danlos patient who 10 years after bilateral TMJ replacement with a stock TMJ replacement device presented with symptoms including headache, local pain, swelling, and erythema. (c and d) After Stage 1 removal of failed stock devices, the stereo laser model (ProtoMED, Westminster, CO) demonstrates loss of temporal-zygomatic bone and the US dime coin-sized fenestration resulting from osteolysis around the loose fossa screw fixation resulting in the perforation of the totally mobile polyethylene fossa component into the middle cranial fossa. TMJ Concepts (Ventura, CA) patient-fitted prosthesis on the patient stereo laser model (e) and implanted (f). The commercially pure titanium mesh backing was designed and manufactured to cover the glenoid fossa fenestration thereby avoiding the need for bone grafting. (g and h) Postoperative plain and orthopantomogram imaging demonstrating the design flexibility of a patient-fitted TMJ replacement system and the adaptation of the components to the host bone. The articulating aspect of the fossa component is ultra-high-molecular weight polyethylene, and therefore it is radiolucent. Case courtesy of Dr. L. Mercuri.

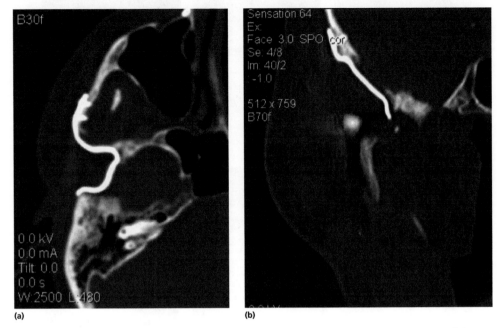

Figure 9.7 Postimplantation axial (a) and coronal (b) CT images demonstrating reconstruction of the glenoid fossa—middle cranial fossa fenestration utilizing the unlimited design potential of a patient-fitted TMJ replacement system. Images for this case were supplied by Dr. Jan Faulk, Chapel Hill, North Carolina.

placement can be planned on the virtual model and the device is designed and incorporated into the planning session. Nerve position and bone thickness are easily visualized, allowing for ideal screw fixation placement. Advantages to this technique allow for precise positioning and measurement of bony segments, as well as simultaneous views in multiple dimensions. Osteotomy or prosthesis design is easily changed or corrected on the virtual model if needed. Finally, unintentional torquing or poor positioning of the contralateral joint can be avoided by overlapping pre- and postoperative images. The preplanned computer model may also be imported into CT-guided surgical software to ensure correct osteotomy site and device positioning intraoperatively or cutting guides can be designed and fabricated. Disadvantages include additional cost of the planning session or software and the absence of a physical model, but it does preclude the "wax-up" stage of the custom implant design.

Combined orthognathic and TMJ prosthetic reconstruction

In cases where a large mandibular advancement or rotation is planned in combination with temporomandibular reconstruction, a custom device may

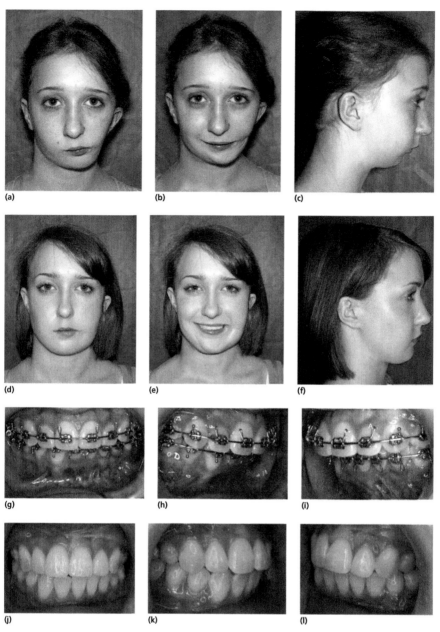

Figure 9.8 (a–c) Fifteen- year-old female diagnosed with (1) left side hemifacial microsomia, (2) absent left TMJ, (3) repaired left transverse facial cleft and cleft palate; (4) maxillomandibular hypoplasia and asymmetry, (5) nasal airway obstruction; (6) class II occlusion; and (7) transverse cant to maxilla, mandible, and occlusal plane. Surgical procedures included the following: Stage 1: (1) left ramus reconstruction with cranial bone grafts, (2) left TMJ reconstruction and mandibular advancement with TMJ Concepts total joint prosthesis, (3) right mandibular sagittal split osteotomy; (4) multiple maxillary osteotomies; (5) fat graft around left TMJ prosthesis; and (6) partial turbinectomies. Surgery Stage 2: (1) AP augmentation osseous genioplasty, (2) fat graft to left mandibular facial area, and (3) reposition otoplasty (left). (d–f). The patient was seen 4 years and 2 months post-surgery demonstrating significantly improved facial balance and function. She has a good Class I skeletal and occlusal relationship and significantly improved facial symmetry. Preoperative occlusion (g–i). Postoperative occlusion (j–l) demonstrating class I relationship. Case courtesy of Dr. Larry Wolford.

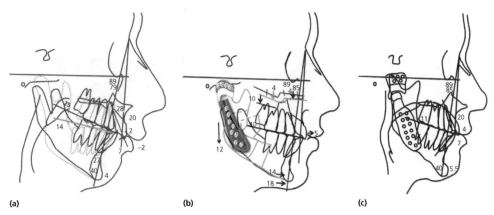

Figure 9.9 Patient from Figure 9.8 with (a) presurgery lateral cephalogram shows the vertical asymmetry and significant retrusion of the mandible and maxilla. (b) Prediction tracing demonstrates the proposed treatment outcome with pogonion advancing 18mm. (c) Four-year 2 month follow-up: radiographic tracing shows the patient maintained good stability of the jaw structures. Case courtesy of Dr. L. Wolford.

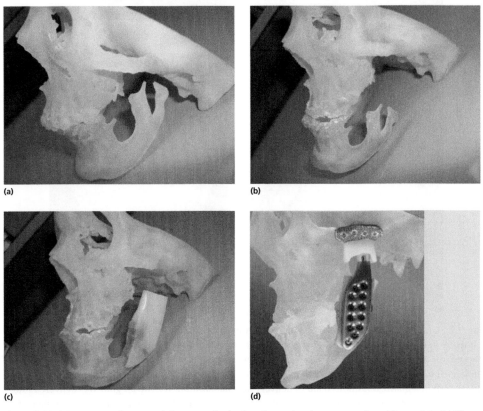

Figure 9.10 (a) 3D stereo laser model accurately depicts the patient's anatomy from Figure 9.8. (b) The mandible was repositioned in a counterclockwise direction with the ramus rotating downward and forward to advance it and transversely level the mandibular occlusal plane, fixed in position with quick cure acrylic. (c) The ramus was reconstructed with cranial bone grafts and the "wax-up" depicted the size and shape of the cranial bone grafts harvested and placed on the lateral and medial sides of the ramus in a "sandwich" design. (d) TMJ Concepts, Inc. manufactured a patient-fitted prosthesis to accommodate the patient's specific anatomical requirements which included the cranial bone grafts to reconstruct the left ramus. Case courtesy of Dr. Larry Wolford.

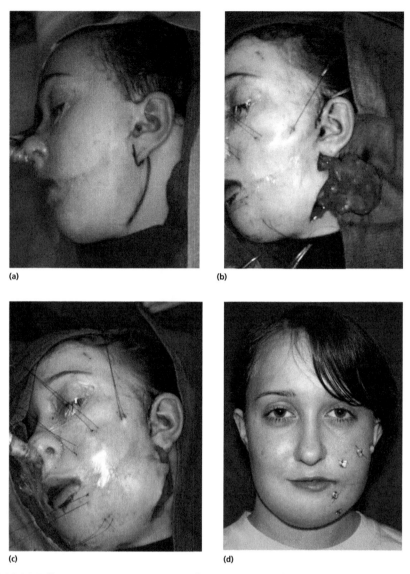

(a)

(b)

(c)

(d)

Figure 9.11 (a) Following Stage 1 surgery (patient from Figure 9.8), there was significant deficiency in soft tissue in the left side of the face. The incision for placement of the augmentation fat graft was marked. (b) An abdominal fat graft was harvested and prepared for transplantation into the left side of the face. Traction sutures were passed at the extension of the tissue pocket dissection and attached to the fat graft in a mattress fashion to aid in delivery and stabilization. (c) The fat graft was delivered into position with the aid of the traction sutures. (d) The patient is seen 1-week post-surgery at the time of suture removal. The cotton balls on the cheek indicate traction sutures to anchor the graft and minimize the tendency for it to "ball-up" in the cheek. Case courtesy of Dr. Larry Wolford.

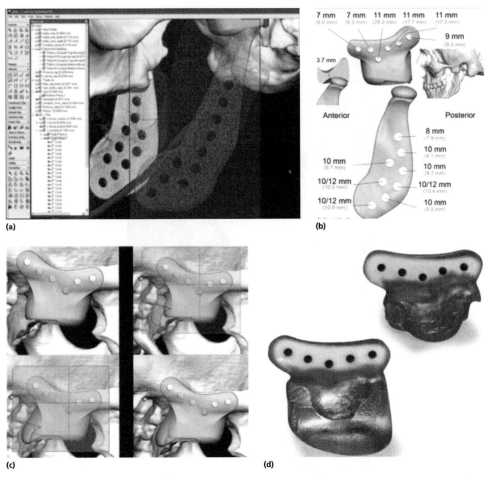

(a)

(b)

(c)

(d)

Figure 9.12 (a) Example of total alloplastic joint surgical planning and design via computer aid modeling (Biomet Microfixation). Utilizing computer design has the added advantage of rapidly producing and comparing alternative designs and treatment plans prior to implementation. (b) Final custom prosthesis design with predetermined screw lengths indicated. (c) Computer-generated fossa design and alternative with anterior eminence extension added. (d) Trial fossa component which can be placed to ensure bone has been adequately reduced, as designed.

be required. Alloplastic reconstruction offers several advantages when used in conjunction with orthognathic surgery, particularly when the TMJ reconstruction is bilateral. The alloplastic device allows for a stable platform for facial reconstruction, as well as the ability to allow for immediate function of the mandible. When a custom device is used, reconstruction of the temporomandibular joint should proceed first, allowing the custom

Fossa prosthesis thickness

Left

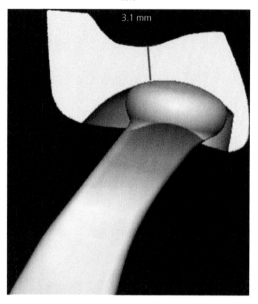

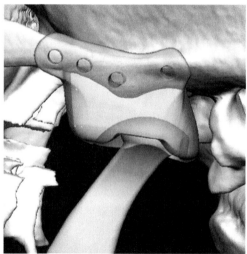

Figure 9.13 Image showing final design and thickness of fossa component in a custom alloplastic total joint replacement. Image courtesy of Biomet Microfixation.

device to act as an intermediate splint. The maxillary osteotomy can then be performed and the maxilla repositioned to the mandible. As in all total temporomandibular joint reconstruction, great care must be taken to avoid intraoral contamination of the prosthetic devices.

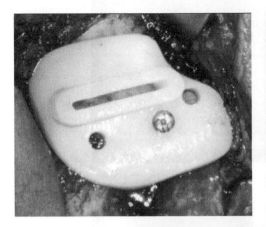
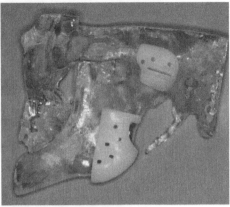

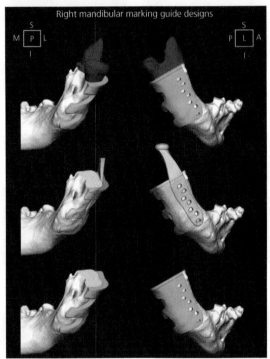

Figure 9.14 Example of custom cutting guides. Once the treatment planning and design is complete, cutting guides can be manufactured to ensure accurate position and angulation of the osteotomies. This optimizes placement and fit of the custom prosthesis, which is often difficult to recapitulate for a custom device intraoperatively. Image courtesy of Biomet Microfixation.

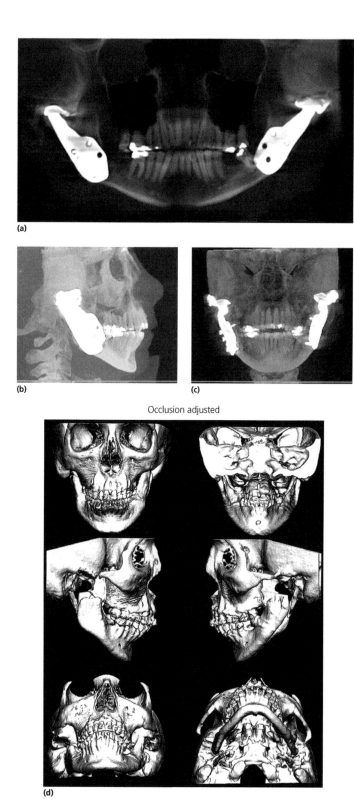

(a)

(b)

(c)

Occlusion adjusted

(d)

Figure 9.15 Images of an infected custom metal-on-metal alloplastic total joint. Note anterior open bite (a–c). (d) Preoperative planned position with malocclusion corrected.

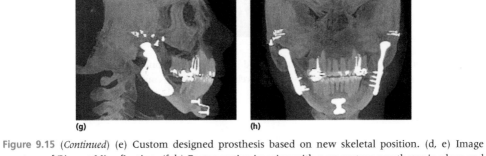

Figure 9.15 (*Continued*) (e) Custom designed prosthesis based on new skeletal position. (d, e) Image courtesy of Biomet Microfixation. (f–h) Postoperative imaging with new custom prostheses in place and malocclusion corrected. Image courtesy of Biomet Microfixation.

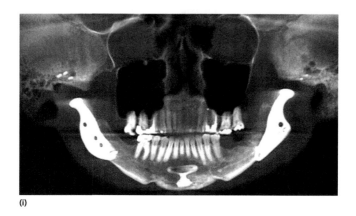

(i)

Splint design

(j)

Figure 9.15 (*Continued*) (i) Postoperative panorex and (j) planned positioning of prosthesis. Note good positioning of custom device and correction of malocclusion. (j) Image courtesy of Biomet Microfixation.

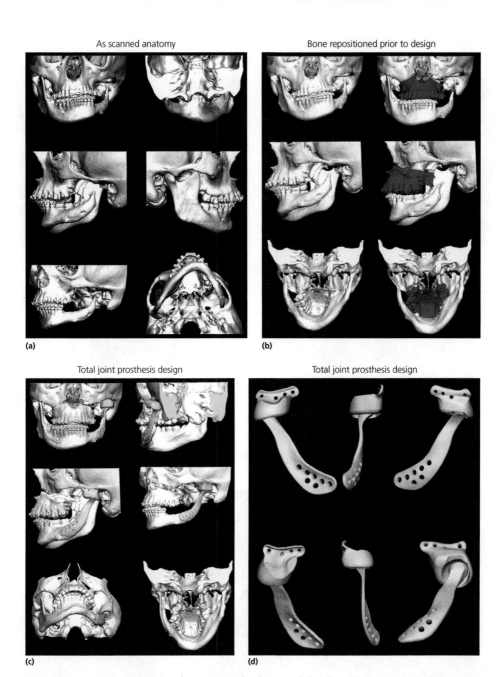

As scanned anatomy

Bone repositioned prior to design

(a)

(b)

Total joint prosthesis design

Total joint prosthesis design

(c)

(d)

Figure 9.16 (a) Preoperative images of a patient with a history of rhabdomyosarcoma, requiring resection, and radiation as a child. Note lack of temporomandibular joint anatomy of the left side. In addition, growth of the patient's midface structures, including the maxilla, was affected. The patient's right side demonstrates normal anatomy and growth. This resulted in moderate skeletal facial asymmetry. (b) Reposition of maxilla (red) into new position in order to correct occlusal cant. Once this is complete, the asymmetric mandible can be repositioned. (c) Computer modeling with maxilla and mandible repositioned to correct the skeletal and occlusal asymmetries. Once the skeletal discrepancies are correct on the computer model, the custom prosthesis can be designed to reconstruct the temporomandibular joint. (d) Images of the custom alloplastic total temporomandibular joint. (a–d) Image courtesy of Biomet Microfixation.

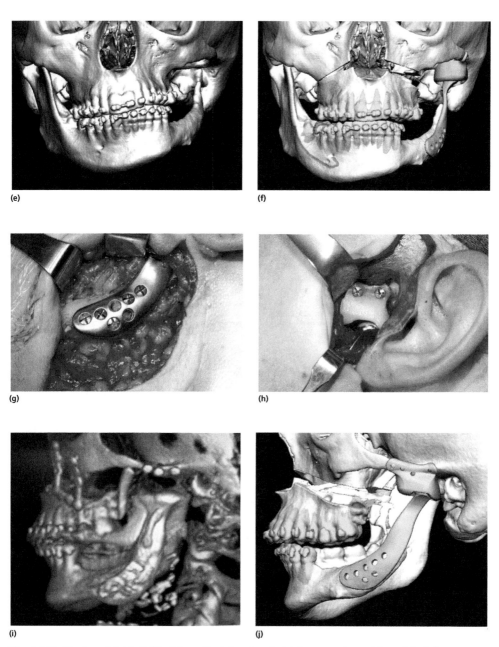

(e)

(f)

(g)

(h)

(i)

(j)

Figure 9.16 (*Continued*) (e) 3-D CT of the patient showing skeletal asymmetry and loss of the left temporomandibular joint. (f) Planned reconstruction to correct facial asymmetry with repositioning of the maxilla with a Lefort 1 osteotomy and repositioning of the mandible with total joint reconstruction. This reconstruction can be accomplished in a single procedure with the use of the custom prosthetic joint, placed first, setting the new position of the mandible. The Lefort 1 osteotomy can then be performed, with the maxilla repositioned to the mandible, correcting the occlusal and facial asymmetry. Intraoperative image of custom prosthesis in place: (g) mandible and (h) fossa component. (i) Postoperative imaging showing custom prosthesis in placed with repositioned maxilla. (j) Preoperative planned surgery.

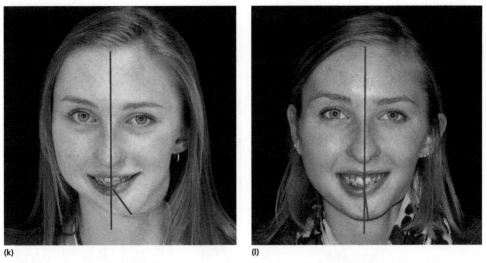

Figure 9.16 (*Continued*) (k) Preoperative image of patient with marked skeletal asymmetry and (l) postoperative image showing improved facial symmetry.

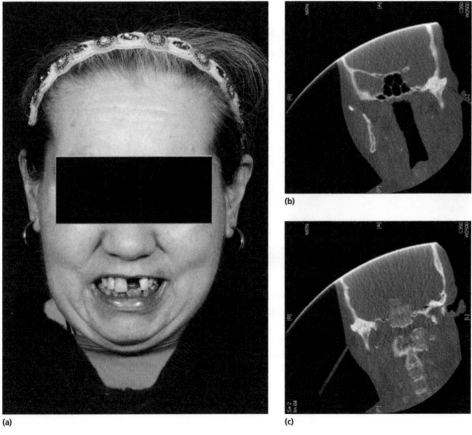

Figure 9.17 (a) The patient at initial presentation with absolute trismus. (b) Patient's left and (c) Patient's Right preoperative CT showing TMJ ankylosis (arrows).

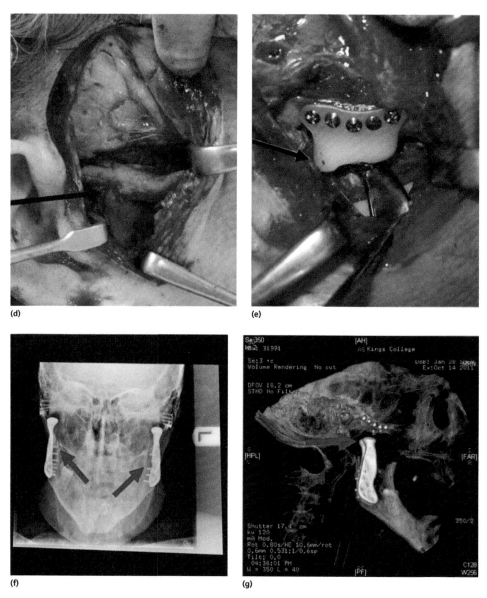

Figure 9.17 (*Continued*) (d) The right TMJ following dissection, showing ankylosis of the joint (arrow). (e) The custom total joint replacement implant in situ (arrow). (e) Postoperative posterior–anterior view of the mandible with the implants in situ (arrows). (f) Postoperative posterior–anterior view of the mandible with the implants in situ (arrows). (g) Postoperative 3D reconstruction showing the implant in place (arrow) (Biomet Microfixation). Images courtesy of Dr. Shaun Matthews.

Further reading

Chandran R. *et al.* (2011) Application of virtual surgical planning for total joint reconstruction with a stock alloplast system. *J Oral Maxillofac Surg*, 69:285.

Granquist EJ, Quinn PD. (2011) Total reconstruction of the temporomandibular joint with a stock prosthesis. *Atlas Oral Maxillofac Surg Clin North Am*, 19:221–232.

Mercuri LG. (2012) Alloplastic temporomandibular joint replacement: rationale for the use of custom devices. *Int J Oral Maxillofac Surg*, 41:1033.

Mercuri LG. *et al.* (2007) A 14-year follow-up of a patient fitted total temporomandibular joint reconstruction system. *J Oral Maxillofac Surg*, 65:1140.

Wolford LM, Dhameja A. (2011) Planning for combined TMJ arthroplasty and orthognathic surgery. *Atlas Oral Maxillofac Surg Clin North Am*, 19:243.

CHAPTER 10

Pathology of the temporomandibular joint

Benign and malignant tumors can affect the structures of the temporomandibular joint. Although tumors are rare compared with disorders of internal derangement and osteoarthritis (see Chapters 4 and 5), the surgeon must always be on the alert for signs of neoplasia. Space-occupying lesions of the joint may present with preauricular swelling, pain, trismus (without deviation on opening or history of joint noise), new-onset malocclusion, or cranial nerve dysfunction. Any of these "red flags" should prompt the surgeon to obtain advanced imaging including an MRI or CT to further evaluate the region. If clinical and radiographic examinations suggest the presence of a tumor, arthroscopic biopsy or open arthrotomy is most helpful to obtain adequate tissue samples. If the mass or tumor is in a difficult region to access surgical, the practitioner may consider obtaining a CT-guided needle biopsy. All the tissues of the temporomandibular joint can serve as a nidus for tumor formation, and the differential diagnosis for a mass in the temporomandibular joint is broad. Rheumatoid and juvenile idiopathic arthritis may also affect the temporomandibular joint and initial management is largely medical. Patients with severe disease, or who are recalcitrant to medical management, may benefit from a surgical intervention.

Rheumatoid arthritis

Advances in medical management of rheumatologic disease has markedly improved the quality of life of these patients and reduced the severity of joint destruction observed, though once joint damaged has occurred, it is largely irreversible. The surgical algorithms for intervention should mirror that used in osteoarthritis, with emphasis on minimizing the number of open arthroplasties and consideration for primary total replacement when severe bony degeneration is evident. In this patient population, surgical management requires close communication with the patient's rheumatologist. Many patients with severe rheumatic conditions will be on immunosuppressive medications.

Atlas of Temporomandibular Joint Surgery, Second Edition. Edited by Peter D. Quinn and Eric J. Granquist.
© 2015 John Wiley & Sons, Inc. Published 2015 by John Wiley & Sons, Inc.
Companion Website: www.wiley.com/go/quinn/atlasTMJsurgery

Table 10.1 Neoplasms of the temporomandibular joint.

Benign tumors and lesions	Malignant tumors
Osteoma	Osteogenic sarcoma
Osteochondroma	Chondrosarcoma
Chondroma	Synovial cell sarcoma
Chondroblastoma	Synovial fibrosarcoma
Giant cell granuloma	Multiple myeloma
Giant cell tumor	Lymphoma
Neurofibroma	Aggressive fibromatosis
Hemangioma	
Arteriovenous malformation	
Synovial chondromatosis	
Osteochondrosis dissecans	
Villonodular synovitis	
Ganglion cyst	

Coordination for the temporary cessation of these medications (e.g., glucocorticoids, disease-modifying antirheumatic drugs and anticytokine medications) in the perioperative period is important to prevent infection and promote healing (see figures 10.13–10.15).

Septic arthritis

Septic arthritis is a rare but potential devastating condition if not promptly recognized and treated. Presently, there have been less than 100 cases reported in the literature, demonstrating both the rarity and difficulty of making a definitive diagnosis. Patients will often present with new temporomandibular or pre-auricular pain, difficulty opening, and preauricular swelling, though these symptoms can be subclinical. The most suggestive physical finding is a new posterior open bite in the absence of recent trauma. A high index of suspicion is

necessary, as culture of the offending organism can be difficult and patients are often prematurely started on antibiotics before a specimen is obtained. Imaging is essential, and a CT scan with contrast is the modality of choice, because it can image soft tissue. MRI can also be utilized but is often difficult to obtain in an acute time frame. Treatment should occur along an emergent timeline. Once lab and imaging data are obtained and continue to support the diagnosis of septic arthritis, cultures should be acquired and antibiotics started. It is often necessary to "washout" the joint and this is best done through arthrocentesis or arthroscopy. If the collection persists or spreads beyond the joint capsule, consideration for open arthrotomy or incision and drainage via a dependent incision location should be considered. Infectious disease consult can be obtained to help guide antibiotic selection and duration (see figures 10.9–10.12).

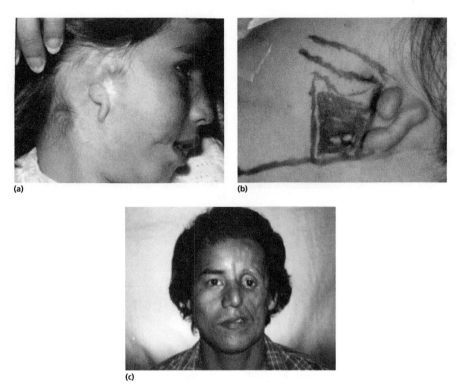

Figure 10.1 (a and b) Hemifacial microsomia with auricular defect. (c) Goldenhar syndrome (oculo-auricular-vertebral syndrome).

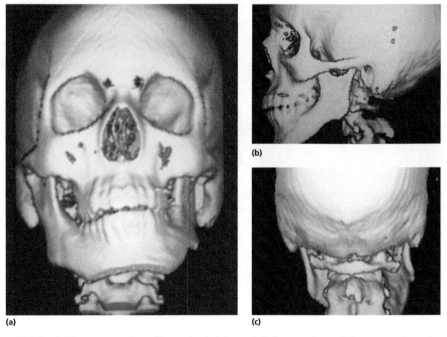

Figure 10.2 (a–c) 3D reconstruction of hypoplastic left condyle from early condylar trauma (age 5).

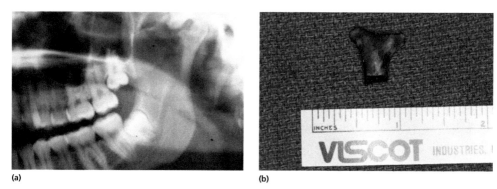

(a)   **(b)**

Figure 10.3 "Hoof" deformity in the condylar head, secondary to condylar trauma during growth, panorex (a) and status post resection (b).

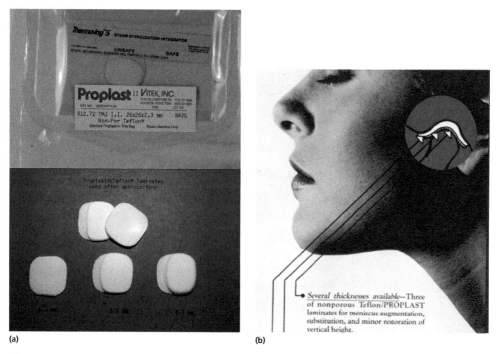

(a)   **(b)**

Figure 10.4 Teflon/proplast implants shown (a) in packaging and (a) demonstration of available sizes and thickness. This implant (b) was used following meniscectomy to maintain height and space between the glenoid fossa and articulating condyle. Poor wear characteristics resulted in foreign body reactions and bone resorption.

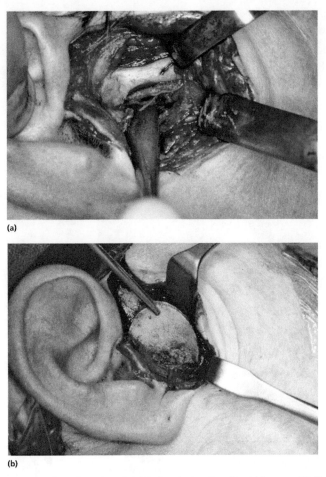

Figure 10.5 (a) Interpositional implant showing Proplast facing the glenoid fossa and Teflon on the inferior articulating surface. (b) Implant being removed with obvious fragmentation of the Proplast-Teflon.

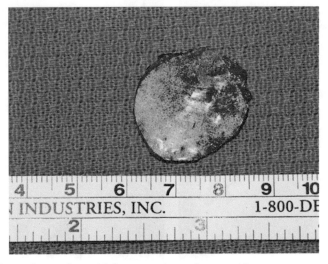

Figure 10.6 Proplast-Teflon implant with fragmentation and wear evident.

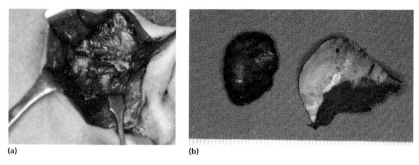

(a)   (b)

Figure 10.7 (a) Giant cell reaction to Proplast-Teflon implant. (b) Fragmentation of implant with associated giant cell tumor.

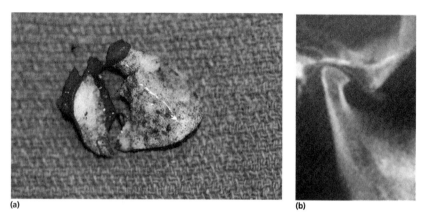

(a)   (b)

Figure 10.8 (a) A perforated Proplast implant. (b) Sagittal CT showing displaced Proplast interpositional implant with irregularities of the condylar head.

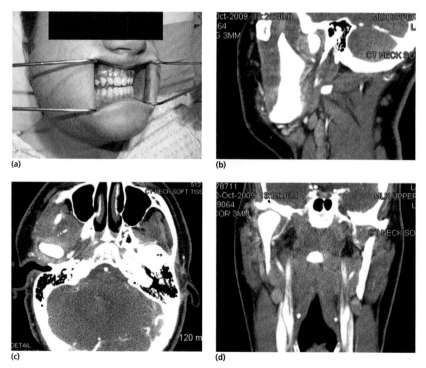

(a)   (b)

(c)   (d)

Figure 10.9 (a) Patient with recent increase in right preauricular swelling, with new posterior open bite and pain with jaw function. (b) Sagittal CT soft-tissue windows with contrast showing rim enhancement of the temporomandibular joint and displacement of the condylar head. (c) Axial and (d) coronal images also showing enhancement of the temporomandibular joint with septic arthritis.

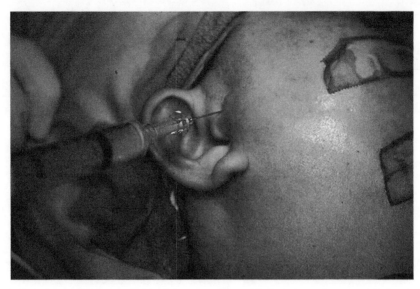

Figure 10.10 Patient with septic arthritis of the temporomandibular joint undergoing initial aspiration of the joint for cytology and culture.

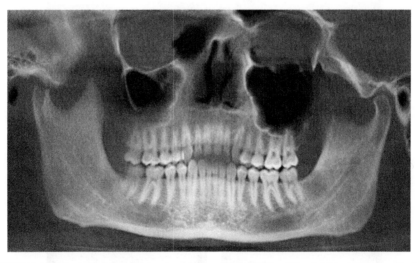

Figure 10.11 Patient 1-week following treatment for septic arthritis of the right temporomandibular joint. Panorex demonstrates acute erosive changes of the condylar head.

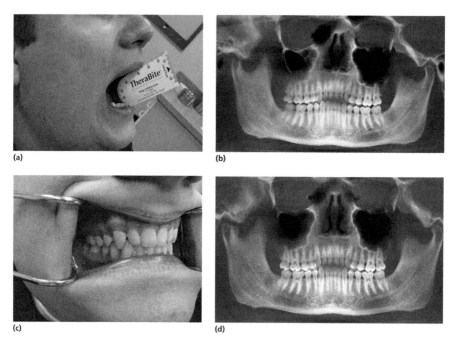

Figure 10.12 Patient from Figure 10.9 1 year later. (a) Patient demonstrating normal pain-free function. (b) One-week postoperative panorex with evidence of severe acute degeneration of the condyle. (c) Return of normal class-1 occlusion. (d) Panorex showing remodeling of the temporomandibular condyle, note cortication of the superior portion of the condyle.

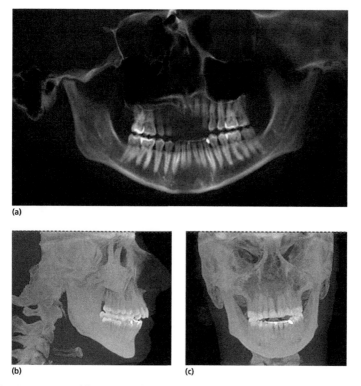

Figure 10.13 (a–c) A 30-year-old patient with a new anterior open bite and progressive joint pain and limited function. Patient was diagnosed with rheumatoid arthritis, which first affected her temporomandibular joints.

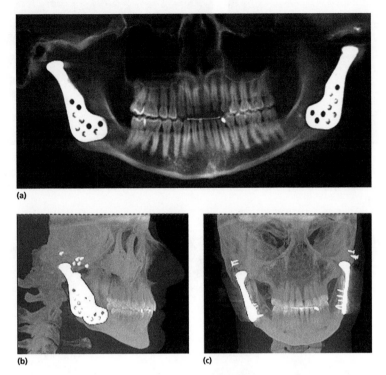

(a)

(b)   (c)

Figure 10.14 (a–c) Patient from Figure 10.13 with rheumatoid arthritis, following bilateral total joint reconstruction and closure of anterior open bite.

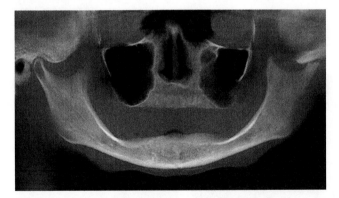

Figure 10.15 Patient with a history of psoriatic arthritis and left joint pain with decreased function. Note severe degeneration of the left joint and loss of joint space when compared to the unaffected right temporomandibular joint.

Benign tumors

If the initial biopsy shows the joint lesion is benign, it may be handled with a standard arthroplasty approach (see Chapter 3). For example, central giant cell granulomas have been known to affect the head of the condyle. They typically appear as solitary, radiolucent lesions of the mandible or maxilla.

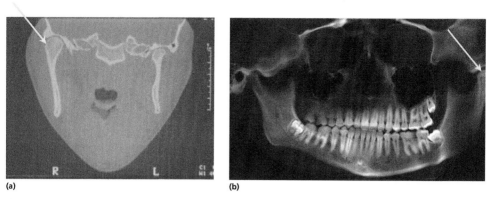

Figure 10.16 (a) Normal condyle on right (arrow) with degenerative condyle on the left contrasted with (b) hemimandibular hypertrophy with enlarged condyle-ramus-body on left (arrow) and normal condyle on right.

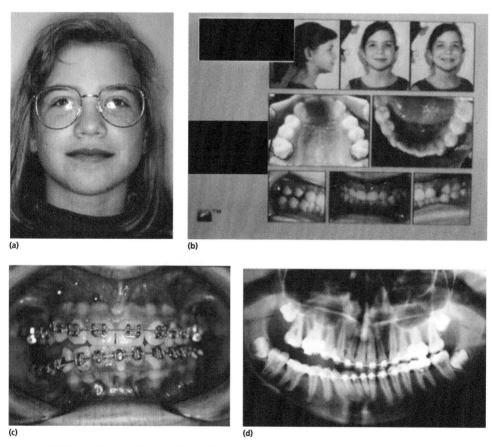

Figure 10.17 (a) A 12-year-old girl with rapid (i.e., over a period of ~4–6 months) onset of a unilateral open bite. (b) Initial orthodontic evaluation prior to onset of rapid unilateral growth. (c) Intraoral occlusal photograph showing marked posterior open bite. (d) Panorex image showing posterior open bite on the right with elongation of the condylar neck, consistent with condylar hyperplasia. Source: Quinn 1998, figure 8.20, p. 235. Reproduced with permission of Elsevier.

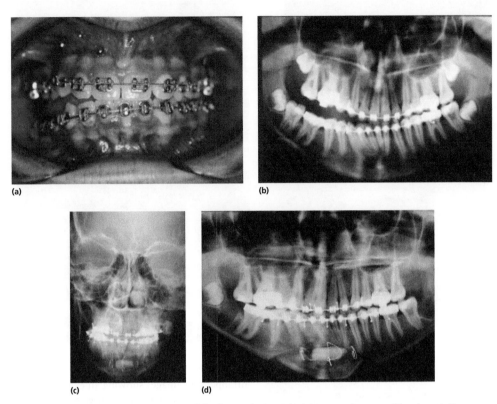

(a)

(b)

(c)

(d)

Figure 10.18 (a and b) Acute-onset condylar hyperplasia with right posterior open bite. (c and d) Post-correction with intraoral vertical subsigmoid osteotomy genioplasty (patient from 10.17).

These lesions tend to involve the jaws anterior to the molar teeth, but they occasionally involve the mandibular ramus and condyle. They usually produce a painless expansion; however, when a space-occupying lesion affects the mandibular condyle, it causes a malocclusion and sometimes a preauricular swelling. Biopsy reveals a stroma of spindle-shaped fibroblasts in the presence of multinucleated giant cells. In the body of the mandible or maxilla, curettage followed by peripheral ostectomy is an acceptable initial approach. When the lesion completely destroys the condylar head, a standard condylectomy can be performed.

Immediate reconstruction can be performed with either autogenous tissues (costochondral graft) or, preferable in the adult patient, an alloplastic prosthesis.

Another benign lesion that requires surgical intervention is synovial chondromatosis. Synovial chondromatosis is a cartilaginous metaplasia that results in the proliferation of abnormal synovia. The hypertrophied synovial tissue produces multiple foci of hyaline cartilage. These cartilaginous nodules can eventually become detached from the synovial membrane and produce "loose bodies" in the joint. These have been referred to in the past as "joint mice." Patients with this

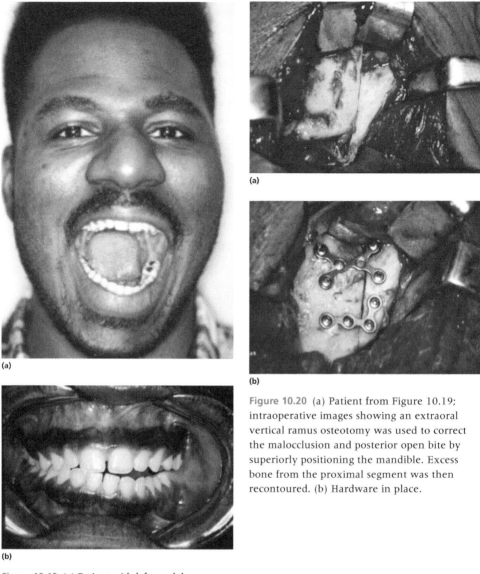

(a)

(b)

Figure 10.20 (a) Patient from Figure 10.19; intraoperative images showing an extraoral vertical ramus osteotomy was used to correct the malocclusion and posterior open bite by superiorly positioning the mandible. Excess bone from the proximal segment was then recontoured. (b) Hardware in place.

(a)

(b)

Figure 10.19 (a) Patient with left condylar hyperplasia (b) Note left open bite.

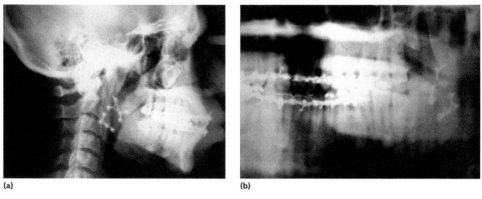

(a)

(b)

Figure 10.21 (a) Lateral cephalometric and (b) panorex (postoperative) of the patient in Figure 10.19.

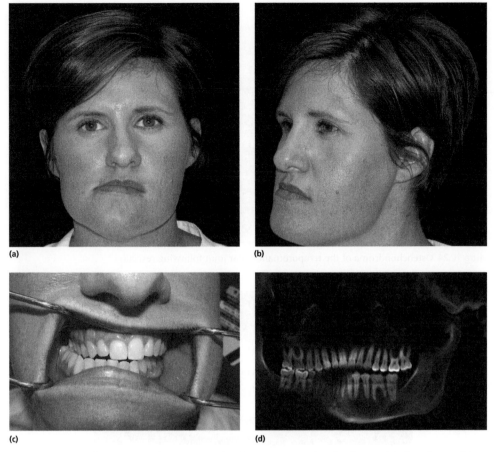

Figure 10.22 (a and b) Patient with progressive facial asymmetry and malocclusion. (c) Note the maxillary midline is congruent with the nose and philtrum. This suggests that the mandibular skeletal asymmetry occurred after the completion of growth. (d) Note the mass (osteochondroma) evident in the left temporomandibular joint.

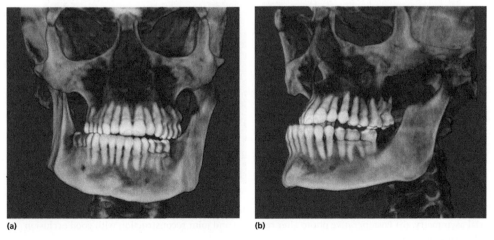

Figure 10.23 (a and b) 3D reconstruction demonstrating large osteochondroma and the mass effect resulting in facial asymmetry and laterognathia.

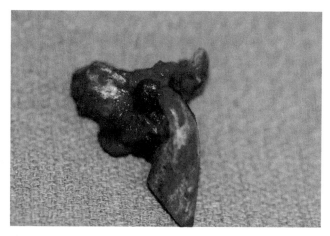

Figure 10.24 Osteochondroma of the temporomandibular joint following resection.

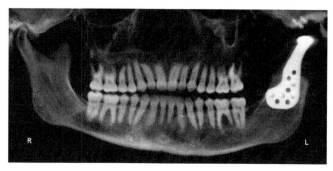

Figure 10.25 Immediate postoperative panorex following resection of an osteochondroma with immediate reconstruction with a stock alloplastic total joint (Biomet Microfixation).

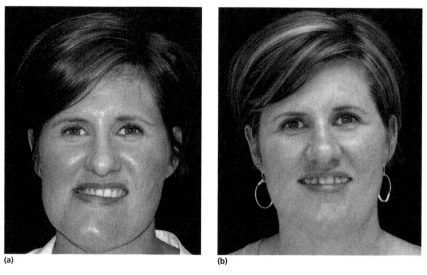

(a)   (b)

Figure 10.26 (a) Preoperative photo of patient with osteochondroma and mass affect with resultant facial asymmetry. (b) Postoperative photo after resection and joint reconstruction with good occlusion and facial symmetry.

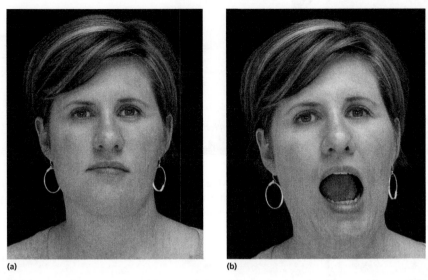

(a) (b)

Figure 10.27 (a) Postoperative image of patient from Figure 10.26 showing chin in midline and (b) with good joint function.

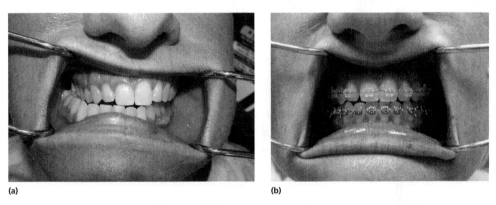

(a) (b)

Figure 10.28 (a) Preoperative occlusion and (b) postoperative occlusion. Note severe midline discrepancy corrected with unilateral joint reconstruction following excision of tumor.

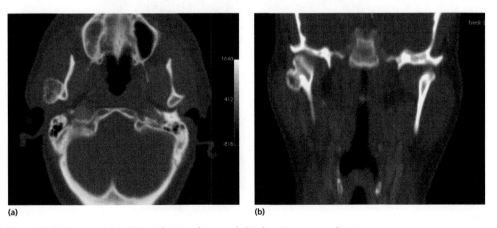

(a) (b)

Figure 10.29 Preoperative CT axial (a) and coronal (b) showing an exophytic osteoma.

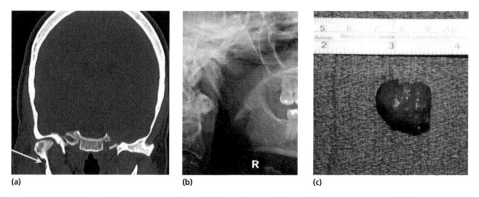

Figure 10.30 (a) Immediate postoperative CT showing excision of benign osteoma of the patient in Figure 10.29 (arrow). The patient was placed in inter-maxillary fixation for two weeks. (b) One-year postoperative panorex showing no recurrence. (c) Osteoma of the temporomandibular joint following excision.

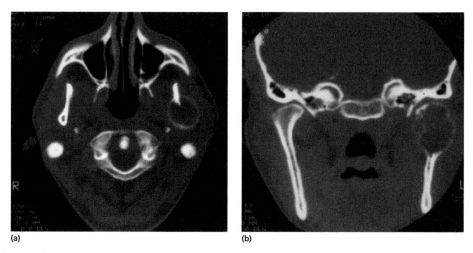

Figure 10.31 (a) Giant cell tumor of the condyle on axial (a) and coronal (b) CT scan of patient.

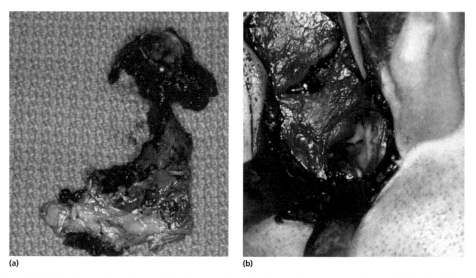

Figure 10.32 (a) Surgical specimen following resection of giant cell tumor from Figure 10.31. (b) Defect present prior to joint reconstruction.

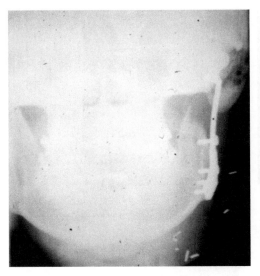 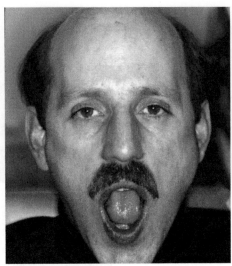

Figure 10.33 Postresection of giant cell tumor with reconstruction plate with condylar head.

condition usually show signs of a space-occupying lesion that causes preauricular swelling, pain, decreased range of motion, and malocclusion. Pressure resorption from collections of these loose cartilaginous bodies can cause perforation of the middle cranial fossa, with leaking of cerebral spinal fluid and resorption of the condyle. Computer tomographic scans and magnetic resonance imaging are extremely helpful in identifying loose bodies in the joint space. The cartilaginous nodules arc radiopaque only if they are sufficiently calcified at the time of the imaging study. The metaplastic synovia can initially be visualized and biopsied by arthroscopy. Once the diagnosis of synovial chondromatosis is made, the treatment is open arthroplasty for removal of the loose bodies and a synovectomy. Although complete removal of all the synovial membrane is impossible, attempts should be made to excise the hypertrophied synovial tissue

wherever possible. A meniscectomy may be necessary to gain access to the metaplastic tissue in advanced cases. In joints where only several loose bodies are identified and the synovial tissue appears to be grossly normal, the loose bodies may be composed of dead cancellous bone and fibrillated cartilage. These characteristics are consistent with osteochondrosis dissecans. This condition does not require an extensive synovectomy and removal of the loose body (or bodies) alone should be sufficient.

A lesion that is classified as benign histologically but extremely aggressive clinically is aggressive fibromatosis. Also called extra-abdominal desmoid, or desmoplastic fibroma, this lesion can occur in the head and neck. The mandible and perimandibular tissues are frequently involved. In some cases, the condition initially presents as trismus because the lesion expands within the masseteric space. This lesion may be

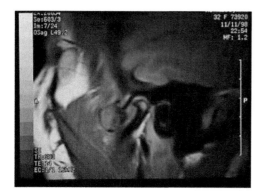 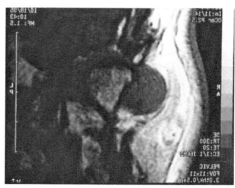

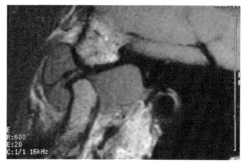

Figure 10.34 Sagittal MRI images of patients with synovial chondromatosis. Note gross distension of the capsule beyond the articular eminence. Often the mass of effect results in degeneration of the condyle, progressive malocclusion, and difficulty with jaw function.

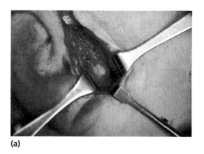 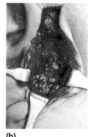 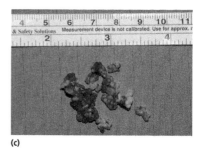

(a) (b) (c)

Figure 10.35 (a) Joint capsule demonstrating gross distension. (b) Joint following entrance into the joint space, note the numerous loose cartilaginous bodies or "joint mice." (c) Specimen of multiple cartilaginous bodies of a patient with synovial chondromatosis.

extremely difficult to diagnose because it is composed of highly differentiated connective tissue with uniform fibroblasts in a collagen stroma. The lesion shows no nuclear atypia, hyperchromatism, or mitotic figures. Diagnosis of aggressive fibromatosis is often based more on the aggressive clinical behavior of the lesion than on histopathologic factors. Recurrences

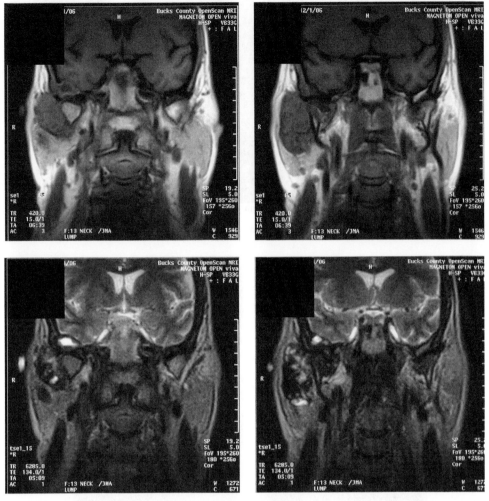

Figure 10.36 Axial MRI showing extensive right joint capsule expansion from synovial chondromatosis.

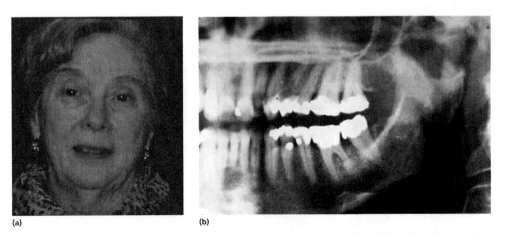

(a)

(b)

Figure 10.37 (a and b) Patient with late-stage synovial chondromatosis with condylar destruction and extension into the base of skull.

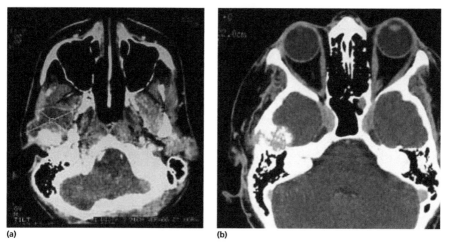

Figure 10.38 (a and b) Base of skull invasion by extensive synovial chondromatosis (patient from Figure 10.37).

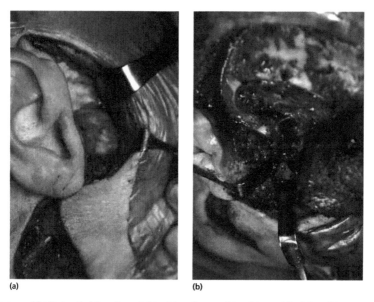

Figure 10.39 (a and b) Extended hemicranial incision for combined lateral facial and intracranial approach to synovial chrondromatosis (patient from Figure 10.37).

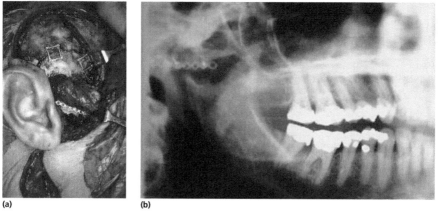

Figure 10.40 Temporal bone flap repositioned after resection of extensive synovial chrondromatosis (a). The inner table of the cranial flap was used to reconstruct the zygomatic arch, note hardware on panorex (b).

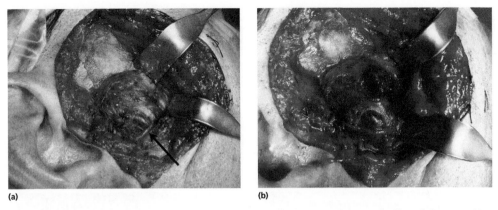

(a)   (b)

Figure 10.41 (a) Exophytic mass of the right temporomandibular joint-pigmented villonodular synovitis (note arrow: temporal branch of the facial nerve displaced by the mass). (b) Pigmented villonodular synovitis. Note the dark pigment of the tumor from hemosiderin.

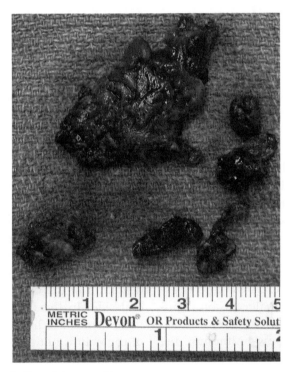

Figure 10.42 Pigmented villonodular synovitis.

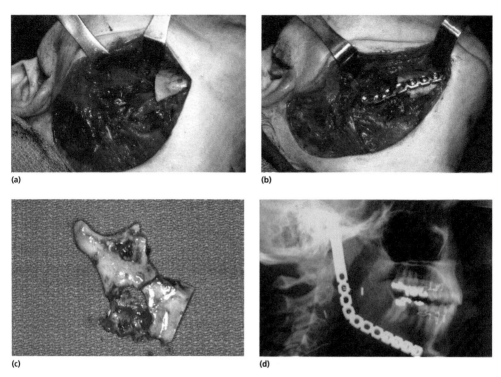

(a)

(b)

(c)

(d)

Figure 10.43 (a) Patient with aggressive fibromatosis with resection of the right mandible to the midbody. (b) Reconstruction plate in place with condylar prosthesis. (c) Surgical specimen with margins. (d) Lateral cephalogram of prosthesis in position.

after conservative surgical excision are reported to be as high as 60%. Therefore the lesion should be approached surgically as a malignancy and adjuvant chemotherapy has effectively been used in recurrent cases.

Although space-occupying benign or malignant lesions can displace the condyle from the fossa and cause asymmetry with malocclusion, condylar hyperplasia can have similar presenting symptoms. Although the actual cause of this disorder is not fully understood, histologic events involve the abnormal presence of hypertrophied hyaline cartilage, which undergoes ossification and results in abnormal growth. In the normal condyle, the articular surface is composed of fibrocartilage that undergoes appositional growth instead of endochondral ossification. Two types of condylar hyperplasia exist. In the type I deformity, or hemi-mandibular elongation, the mandible is asymmetric with deviation of the chin to the contralateral side. In the type II deformity, or hemi-mandibular hypertrophy, deviation of the chin is not a prominent feature, but a marked vertical open bite is present on the side of the hyperplasia. Condylar hyperplasia is not a true neoplasia but actually a self-limiting disorder. Radionuclide bone scans with technetium 99 m can be helpful in differentiating between active and inactive disorders. Some researchers favor the use of a high condylar shave to remove the zone of abnormal tissue if the disorder is diagnosed early in its active stages. Removal of only 5 or 6 mm of the most superior condylar surface is usually adequate and condylectomy is unnecessarily aggressive. Surgeons sometimes must perform a recontouring of the inferior border and angle of the mandible in conjunction with this procedure to address the inferior component of the mandibular asymmetry. When the bone scan shows that the process is inactive, orthognathic procedures such as an intraoral vertical sub-sigmoid osteotomy can be useful in closing the open bite while maintaining a functional joint articulation. In severe cases, condylectomy with immediate prosthetic joint replacement can be indicated.

Foreign body reactions

Although foreign body reaction to alloplastic implants is not usually considered an inherent pathology of the temporomandibular joint, it is worth mentioning. In the early 1980s, initial success was reported with a teflon-proplast implant used as a disk replacement. Before that, block Silastic was the alloplastic material most often used after gap arthroplasty. In the mid 1980s, clinicians began to report biomechanical failure of Teflon-Proplast interpositional implants, causing condylar resorption, pain, and malocclusion. Since that time

the oral and maxillofacial surgery community has become aware of the pathology of polymeric debris in the temporomandibular joint. Proplast (polytetraflouroethylene) had been used as an onlay implant for chin and zygomatic arch augmentation. Used in that context, it formed a fibrous encapsulation and was not widely known to cause any pathologic response. Unfortunately, when placed in a loaded joint, the material can fragment. This point is extremely important because it is clearly the size of the polymeric particle that determines the aggressiveness of the foreign body reaction. Particles small enough to undergo phagocytosis stimulate a multi-nucleated giant cell reaction that can cause marked destruction of the temporomandibular joint. When used for permanent joint implantation, silicone rubber has also been known to cause a foreign-body giant cell reaction with articular erosion. The reaction does not appear to be as aggressive as those associated with the interpositional Proplast implants. (In light of these findings, most surgeons recommend the removal of Teflon-Proplast implants.) If asymptomatic patients decide against this approach, they should receive regular clinical and radiographic examinations to ensure that no adverse reactions are taking place. When silicone sheeting is used as a temporary replacement (6–8 weeks), it stimulates a connective tissue encapsulation. This has been very successful in preventing the formation of fibrous adhesions after meniscoplasty or meniscectomy.

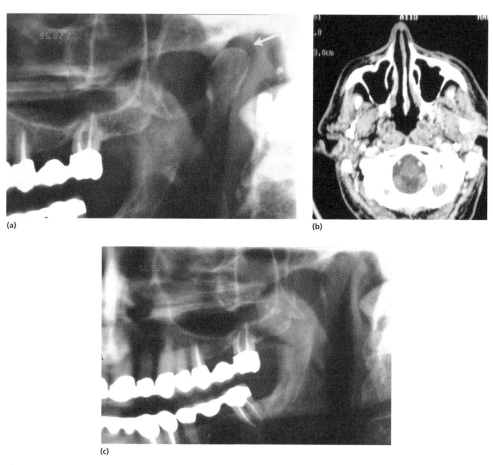

Figure 10.44 (a) Preoperative panorex showing displaced condyle (arrow) by a space-occupying lesion in the glenoid fossa. (b) Axial CT scan showing infiltrating soft tissue lesion of the left temporomandibular joint with erosion into the skull base. (c) Panorex following mass debulking with condyle seated in a more physiologic position. The lesion was diagnosed as aggressive fibromatosis.

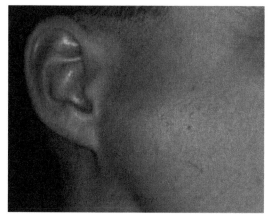

Figure 10.45 Palpable exophytic mass of the right temporomandibular joint. Fine-needle aspiration confirmed osteogenic sarcoma.

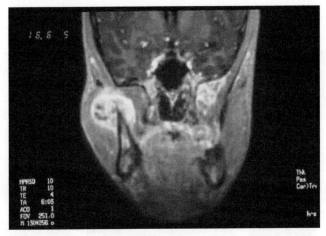

Figure 10.46 Coronal MRI depicting a large mass of the condylar head displacing the condylar head, medial pterygoid, and masseter found to be an osteogenic sarcoma.

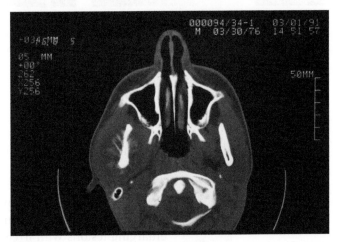

Figure 10.47 Axial CT (bone windows) of the patient from Figure 10.45 showing radiating irregular spicules of bone producing a "sun-ray" appearance (osteogenic sarcoma).

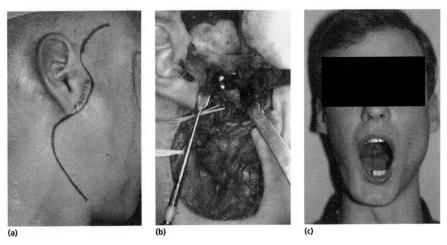

(a) (b) (c)

Figure 10.48 (a) An extended parotid-type incision with temporal extension for resection of the osteogenic sarcoma. Note the preauricular incision which was used for the biopsy. (b) Mass excised with reconstruction plate and condylar head component in place. A sternocleidomastoid flap was rotated anteriorly and superiorly to help with wound coverage. (c) Patient postoperative showing good function.

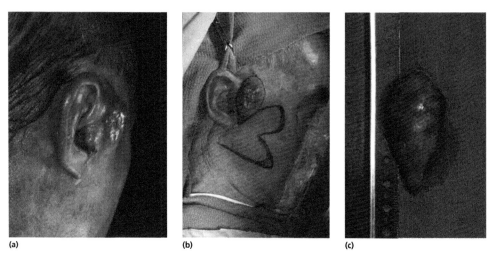

(a)   (b)   (c)

Figure 10.49 (a) A 55-year-old man with an exophytic preauricular mass. (b) Tumor excision with bilobed closure. (c) Excised mass diagnosed as metastatic adenocarcinoma secondary to a colon tumor.

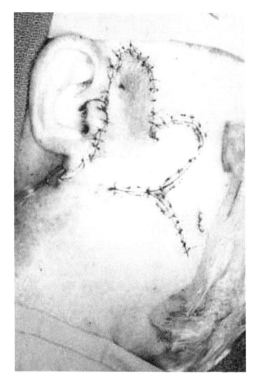

Figure 10.50 Bilobed closure following resection of the preauricular mass (adenocarcinoma).

Malignant tumors

The malignant lesions affecting the temporomandibular joint can originate in various articular tissues. Osteosarcoma, chondrosarcoma, and synovial sarcoma have been reported. Painful, rapidly enlarging lesions with irregular borders suggest malignant neoplasms. Erosion into the middle ear and base of the skull may have occurred at the time of initial diagnosis. The clinician must be especially careful in differentiating chondrosarcoma from synovial chondromatosis because these conditions are frequently mistaken for one another. Chondrosarcomas usually appear as lytic lesions with random areas of calcification. Mesenchymal chondrosarcoma is a highly malignant variant of chondrosarcoma that requires a radical surgical excision and often metastasizes to lung or bone.

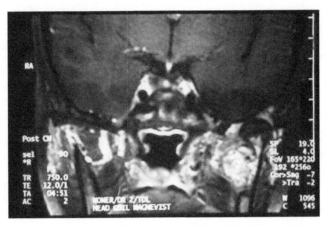

Figure 10.51 MRI showing mass on the medial aspect of the condyle shown to be an osteogenic sarcoma in a pediatric patient.

Approximately 5% of osteosarcomas occur in the jaws. They appear most frequently in men between 30 and 40 years of age. Like osteochondromas, they commonly present as preauricular swelling with painful, rapidly enlarging lesions. Paresthesia may occur secondary to a compression neuropathy involving the inferior alveolar nerve. Variants of osteosarcoma that may affect the temporomandibular joint are the osteoblastic, fibroblastic, and chondroblastic osteosarcomas. They tend to initially appear as lytic lesions. Common sites for metastasis are the lung and brain. Osteosarcomas are best treated by radical wide excision, and radiotherapy and chemotherapy are reserved for recurrences. (Chondrosarcomas are relatively radioresistant.)

The most common malignancy affecting skeletal bones is metastatic carcinoma. Although only 1% of malignant neoplasms metastasize to the jaws, the most common sites for metastasis are secondary to primary carcinomas in the breast, kidney, lung, colon, prostate, and thyroid gland. Unexplained paresthesia, loosening of teeth, spontaneous bone pain, and pathologic fracture can be presenting symptoms of metastatic carcinoma. Ill-defined radiolucent lesions that do not respond to extraction or endodontic therapy demand immediate biopsy. Initial diagnosis of a metastatic lesion requires a complete workup to identify the primary site of malignancy.

Further reading

Alexander WN, Nagy WW. (1973) Gonococcal arthritis of the temporomandibular joint: report of a case. *Oral Surg Oral Med Oral Pathol*, 36:809.

Barnes L. (1985) *Surgical pathology of the head and neck*, vol 2, Marcel Dekker, New York.

Bell WH, editor. (1992) *Modern practice in orthognathic and reconstructive surgery*, vol 2, WB Saunders, Philadelphia.

Cai XY. *et al.* (2010) Septic arthritis of the TMJ. *J Oral Maxillofac Surg*, 68:731.

Cohen S, Quinn P. (1988) Facial trismus and myofascial pain associated with infections and malignant disease: report of five cases. *Oral Surg Oral Med Oral Pathol*, 65:538.

Dahlin D, Unni K. (1986) *Bone tumors,* ed 4, vol 111, Charles C Thomas, Springfield.

Daspit C, Spetzler R. (1989) Synovial chondromatosis of the temporomandibular joint with intracranial extension: case report. *J Neurosurg,* 70:121.

DeBoom G. *et al.* (1985) Metastatic tumors of the mandibular condyle: review of the literature and report of a case. *Oral Surg Oral Med Oral Pathol,* 60:512.

Eisenbud I. *et al.* (1988) Central giant cell granuloma of the jaws: experiences in the management of 37 cases. *J Oral Maxillofac Surg,* 46:376.

Feinerman DM, Piecuch JF. (1993) Long-term retrospective analysis of twenty-three Proplast-Teflon temporomandibular joint interpositional implants. *J Oral Maxiliofac Surg,* 22:11.

Garrington G, Collett W. (1988a) Chondrosarcoma I: a select literature review. *J Oral Pathol,* 17:1.

Garrington G, Collett W. (1988b) Chondrosarcoma II: chondrosarcoma of the jaws: analysis of 37 cases. *J Oral Pathol,* 17:12.

Gorlin R, Goldman H. (1970) *Thomas's oral pathology,* ed 6, Mosby, St. Louis.

Granquist EJ, Quinn PD. (2011) Total reconstruction of the temporomandibular joint with a stock prosthesis. *Atlas Oral Maxillofac Surg Clin North Am,* 19:221–232.

Hackney F. *et al.* (1991) Chondrosarcoma of the jaws: clinical findings, histopathology and treatment. *Oral Surg Oral Med Oral Pathol,* 71:139.

Kaban L. (1990) *Pediatric oral and maxillofacial surgery,* WB Saunders, Philadelphia.

Kochan E. (1963) Reparative giant cell granuloma. *J Oral Surg,* 21:390.

Loftus MJ. *et al.* (1986) Osteochondroma of the mandibular condyles. *Oral Surg,* 61:221.

Norman J. *et al.* (1988) Synovial osteochondrosis of the temporomandibular joint: an historical review with presentation of 3 cases. *J Craniomaxillofac Surg,* 16:212.

Papavsiliou A. *et al.* (1983) Benign conditions of the temporomandibular joint: a diagnostic dilemma. *Br J Oral Surg,* 21:222.

Ruben MM. *et al.* (1989) Metastatic carcinoma of the mandibular condyle presenting as temporomandibular joint syndrome. *J Oral Maxillofac Surg,* 478:511.

Ryan DE. (1989) Alloplastic implants in the temporomandibular joint. *Oral Maxillofac Clin North Am,* 1:427.

Schellhas KP. *et al.* (1988) Permanent Proplast temporomandibular joint implant: MR imaging of destructive complications. *AJR Am J Roentgenol,* 151:731.

Schulte WC, Rhyne RR. (1969) Synovial chondromatosis of the temporomandibular joint. *Oral Surg,* 28:906.

Sidebottom AJ, Salha R. (2013) Management of the temporomandibular joint in rheumatoid disorders. *Br J Oral Maxillofac Surg,* 51:191.

Spagnoli D, Kent JN. (1992) Multicenter evaluation of Proplast-Teflon temporomandibular joint disc implant. *Oral Surg Oral Med Oral Pathol,* 74:411.

Stewart J. (1989) Benign non-odontogenic tumors. In *Oral pathology: clinical-pathologic correlations* (Eds J Regezi and J Sciubba). WB Saunders, Philadelphia.

Wagner JD, Mosby EL (1990) Assessment of Proplast-Teflon disc replacement. *J Oral Maxillofac Surg,* 48:1140.

Waldron CA. (1985) Fibro-osseous lesions of the jaws. *J Oral Maxillofac Surg,* 43:249.

Zachariades N. (1989) Neoplasms metastatic to the mouth, jaws, and surrounding tissues. *J Craniomaxillofac Surg,* 17:283.

CHAPTER 11

Complications

Temporomandibular joint (TMJ) surgery including arthroscopy and arthrotomy, like all other types of surgery, can result in complications. The complications can be transient or long term.

Nerve injury

Injuries to the branches of cranial nerves V and VII are untoward, though acceptable risks in TMJ surgery. Arthroscopy is less likely than arthrotomy to cause permanent malfunction manifesting as an interference with facial expression and cosmetic deformity. The reported incidence of facial nerve injury following TMJ surgery ranges from 1 to 25% and is typically transient in nature, resolving within 3–6 months. Causes of neuropraxia include edema, excessive flap retraction forces, electrocautery, inadvertent suture ligation, or clamping of tissues.

Surgical approaches to the TMJ have been designed to afford the most protection to the facial nerve. Regardless of the surgical approach that is utilized, facial nerve injury is always a risk. The temporal and zygomatic branches of the facial nerve are most prone to injury, presenting, respectively, as a loss of ability to raise one's eyebrow and wrinkle their forehead or close their eye completely. Prevention of disruption of the branches of the facial nerve requires a comprehensive knowledge of the anatomy and meticulous surgical dissection. Factors that can increase the risk of nerve damage include use of improper surgical technique or abnormal joint anatomy as a result of a congenital abnormality, trauma, tumor, or multiple previous surgeries.

Postsurgical palsy of the temporal branch of the facial nerve manifests as an inability to raise the eyebrow and ptosis of the brow. Complications from this nerve injury are largely cosmetic but ptosis of the brow may interfere with peripheral vision. Injury to the zygomatic branch of the facial nerve is more concerning and results in paresis of the orbicularis oculi. This injury may require temporary patching of the eye to prevent corneal desiccation and abrasion. In addition, patients should be prescribed ophthalmic drops including artificial tears for daytime use and a

Atlas of Temporomandibular Joint Surgery, Second Edition. Edited by Peter D. Quinn and Eric J. Granquist.
© 2015 John Wiley & Sons, Inc. Published 2015 by John Wiley & Sons, Inc.
Companion Website: www.wiley.com/go/quinn/atlasTMJsurgery

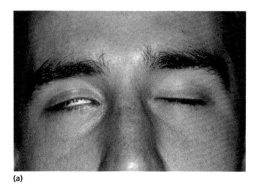
(a)

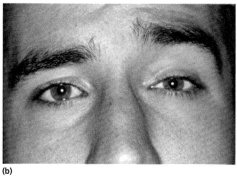
(b)

Figure 11.1 (a) Paresis of the zygomatic branch of the facial nerve (CN VII). The patient has weakness of the orbicularis oculi and hence is unable to close his eye. This can result in severe drying of the cornea, with desiccation and corneal abrasion. (b) Paresis of the temporal branch of the facial nerve (CN VII). The patient has weakness of the frontalis muscle so he is unable to wrinkle his forehead and raise his eyebrow. Source: Quinn 1998, figure 3.29, p 48. Reproduced with permission of Elsevier.

petrolatum-based ointment for use at night to maintain moisture. Permanent nerve damage may necessitate tarsorrhaphy before a more permanent functional approach, such as implantation of a gold weight for gravity-assisted closure of the upper lid is indicated. Galvanic stimulation can be helpful in speeding recovery after a neuropraxia-type injury and should be considered.

Injury to the trigeminal nerve branches (the infraorbital nerve, the inferior alveolar nerve, and lingual nerve) is less common in TMJ surgery. Both preauricular and endaural approaches to the joint, by nature, interfere with auriculotemporal innervation. A more serious injury to the inferior alveolar nerve can occur from instruments used to clamp the mandible in order to distract the condyle inferiorly. It can also be damaged during condylectomy or screw placement, used to fixate mandibular implants. The prognosis for recovery from these injuries is less predictable.

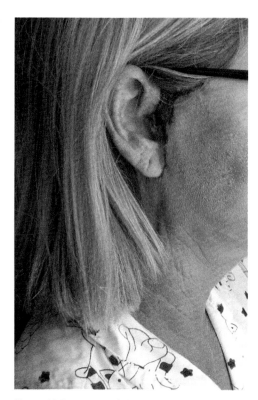

Figure 11.2 Necrosis of the skin flap following a hematoma with an endaural approach to the temporomandibular joint.

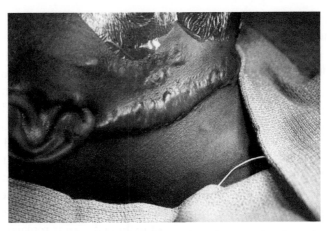

Figure 11.3 Postsurgical keloid sometimes referred to as a keloid scar is a firm heaped-up scar that rises quite abruptly above the rest of the skin. It usually has a smooth top and a pink or purple color. Keloids are irregularly shaped and tend to enlarge progressively. Unlike scars, keloids do not subside over time.

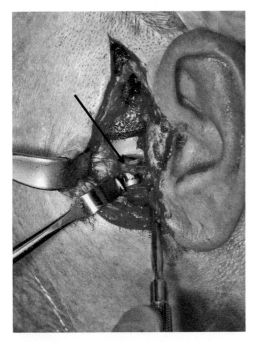

Figure 11.4 Periprosthetic soft tissue (arrow). The patient had extensive pain associated with the implant. Excision of the soft tissue revealed a surgical neuroma, with subsequent marked improvement in pain symptoms.

Hemorrhage

Bleeding is most often encountered from the middle meningeal artery, internal maxillary artery, masseteric artery or bleeding from the lateral pterygoid muscles. Identification and ligation of the severed vessel is clearly preferred but often difficult. Several hemostatic agents should be available to help with bleeding, particularly since many of these vessels can be difficult to identify through the standard approaches or small oozing may persist from the muscle or bone osteotomies. It is essential to have a hemostatic field prior to closure to prevent hematoma formation and fibrosis and scarring. Thrombin, collagen, or tissue adhesives may be utilized to decrease bleeding. For more brisk bleeds, which are difficult to control, access to the external carotid artery is possible through the retromandibular incision.

In a standard neck approach to the external carotid artery, it is important to identify at least three branches to ensure proper identification of the external carotid artery before it is ligated. In addition, ligation of this artery should occur above the level of the facial artery to adequately decrease flow. Lastly, interventional radiology may be considered to identify and occlude a bleeding vessel via embolization.

Heterotopic bone formation

Heterotopic bone formation (HTBF) and reankylosis can be a difficult problem, particularly in the multioperated patient. In addition to excessive bone formation, often extensive scarring makes achieving acceptable maximal incisal openings difficult. HTBF is an early event after surgery involving joint spaces. Most cases have occurred within 2–3 months of trauma or surgery. HTBF can be associated with significant pain and restricted joint movement.

Several methods to combat HTBF have been addressed in the orthopedic literature. This includes nonsteroidal anti-inflammatory medication (indomethacin) and the use of low-dose postsurgical radiation. Reported regimens include 10 Gy in five fractionated daily doses in the immediate postoperative period. Wolford reported the use of autogenous fat grafting around the prosthetic joint to prevent bone formation and scarring. In this case series of 37 joints, no patient grafted with fat formed heterotopic bone, compared to 35% of the controls.

Infection

Postsurgical infections, in TMJ surgeries when an implant was not placed, occur infrequently. With total TMJ replacement, immediate infection of the components is atypical. Late infection can occur and is associated with biofilm formation. These are matrix-enclosed, surface-associated communities that are protected from host defenses and antibiotics. Biomaterial-associated infections of orthopedic joint replacements are the second most common cause of implant failure.

The bacteria that are most commonly isolated from biofilm-infected medical devices are *Staphylococcus epidermidis*. *Staphylococcus aureus*, *Pseudomonas aeruginosa*, the *Enterococcus* species, and infrequently, the Candida species are also encountered. Broad-spectrum antibiotics should be used empirically, followed by culture and microanalysis of the explanted prosthesis. The utilization of aseptic technique, perioperative

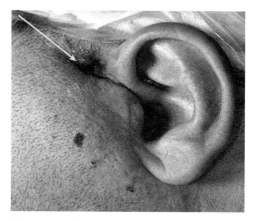

Figure 11.5 Chronic fistula (arrow) associated with an infected prosthetic implant.

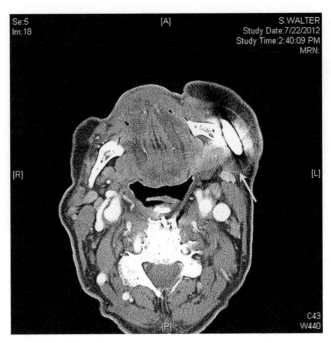

Figure 11.6 CT scan of ring-enhancing collection around the left mandibular ramus. Postoperative infections in TMJ surgeries are almost exclusively associated with alloplastic implants. Late infection is most common and is associated with biofilm formation.

antibiotics, and meticulous surgery can minimize the occurrence of device-related biofilm. This includes thorough irrigation of the external auditory canal with an antibiotic-impregnated solution and fastidious attention to separation of extra-oral and intra-oral fields. Other maneuvers such as soaking prosthetic devices in an antibiotic solution prior to implantation should be considered.

Late effects of condylar fractures

Condylar fractures are common injuries, comprising approximately 25% of all mandibular fractures. In the adult population, condylar fractures result mostly from motor vehicle accidents. Assaults, falls, accidents at work, and trauma during sporting events comprise other mechanisms. In children, falls and bicycle accidents account for the majority of condylar fractures, followed by motor vehicle accidents.

With a better knowledge of the anatomy of the TMJ apparatus, and improved surgical techniques, open reduction and internal fixation of condylar fractures can lead to quicker and more precise return of preoperative function with improved facial symmetry and overall esthetics, when compared to earlier nonsurgical techniques. Of particular concern with fractures

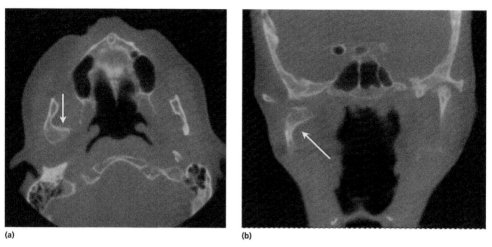

(a)   (b)

Figure 11.7 Axial (a) and coronal (b) CT scan showing malunion of a displaced, untreated right condylar fracture (arrow). Note the differences in vertical height between the two condyles on the axial and coronal CTs. Asymmetry after condylar fracture is common and is influenced by the degree of displacement. This is exemplified as a decrease in mandibular ramus height resulting in a shorter lower facial third on the fracture side. Optimally, anatomic reapproximation of the condylar fracture segments and reestablishment of a stable and reproducible occlusion should be accomplished with open rigid-fixation techniques.

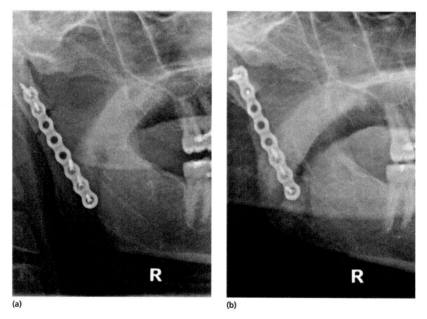

(a)   (b)

Figure 11.8 Panorex X-ray of immediate postreduction (a) and following blunt facial trauma (b). Screw failure occurred at the bone interface, resulting in displacement of the proximal segment. Note the disruption of the posterior border of ramus at the level of the fracture at the condylar neck.

involving the TMJ are the complications including ankylosis, loss of facial height, trismus, traumatic arthritis, and decreased or asymmetric growth in adolescent patients. Ankylosis, though rare, is more often seen in capsular-burst fractures, condylar fractures associated with symphyseal fracture and saggital condylar fractures when lateral displacement occurs. Trismus is often secondary to muscle injury and an exam under anesthesia can aid in the diagnosis muscle-versus-mechanical obstruction. Patients with bilateral TMJ fractures and loss of vertical dimension necessitate an open reduction to restore adequate height.

Identification of condylar fractures in pediatric patients can be difficult. Children are often frightened in the emergency room setting and less able to convey subjective symptoms of their injury. Younger patients (up to ~12 years of age) can exhibit a complete and rapid restitution of their condyle anatomy with conservative therapy. A brief period of intermaxillary fixation (7–10 days) is often sufficient to allow adequate healing and minimize the risk of ankylosis. The period of fixation should be adjusted for the age of the child, with younger patients requiring less time for immobilization. Close supervision is an absolute requirement to monitor facial growth. Early referral to an orthodontist should be considered.

Materials failure

Unfortunately, the history of alloplastic TMJ reconstruction has been characterized by multiple highly publicized failures based on inappropriate design, lack of attention to biomechanical principles, and ignorance of what already had been documented in the orthopedic literature.

(*Quinn First edition*)

Mercuri and Anspach published a comprehensive review of the various types of materials failure including (i) foreign body reaction with implant loosening, (ii) component fracture, and (iii) fixation failure.

The Kent-Vitek Prosthesis (VK-I) was one of the first total TMJ prostheses that was extensively used in the United States. This system originally consisted of a bilaminate glenoid fossa implant. Its articulating surface was Teflon®-coated fluoroethyl polyethylene (FEP) and its tissue-side surface was polytetrafluoroethylene (PTFE, Proplast®). The PTFE could be carved to fit the individual glenoid fossa. The condylar component was made of chrome-cobalt with a PTFE liner on the inner surface of the ramal flange. In 1986, the fossa component was modified, consisting of an ultra-high-molecular-weight polyethylene (UHMWPE) outer layer and a PTFE-hydroxyapatite inner layer. Shortly thereafter, various authors reported bony resorption and foreign body reaction with giant cells in TMJs implanted with PTFE.

Currently, there are three FDA-approved total TMJ replacement systems available: (i) the Christensen TMJ Prosthesis System® (TMJ Implants, Inc.), (ii) the TMJ Concepts® Prosthesis, and (iii) the Biomet Microfixation TMJ Replacement System®. The TMJ Concepts Prosthesis and the Biomet Microfixation TMJ Replacement

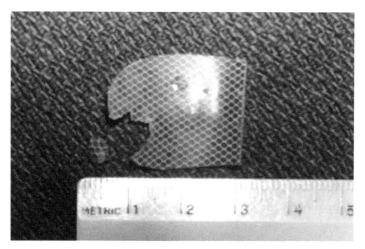

Figure 11.9 Dacron-reinforced silicone sheet showing wear and fragmentation.

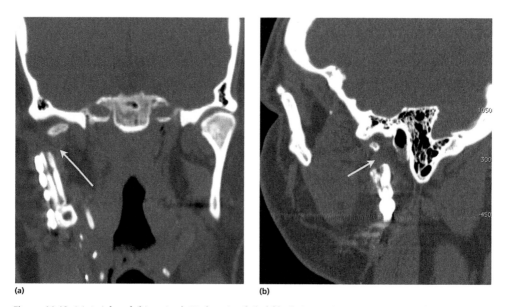

(a)   (b)

Figure 11.10 (a) Axial and (b) sagittal CT showing failed fibula (arrow) reconstruction with resorption to the level of the reconstruction plate.

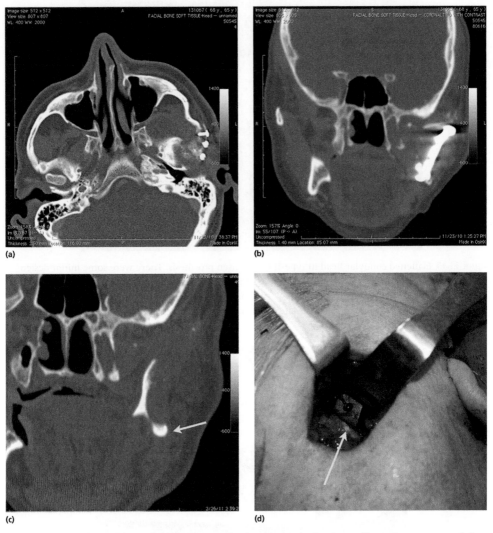

(a)

(b)

(c)

(d)

Figure 11.11 Axial (a) and coronal (b) CT scan showing foreign-body giant cell reaction status post left TMJ reconstruction with a Kent-Vitek prosthesis. (c) Coronal CT scan and (d) intraoperative view. Giant cell reaction with extensive bony erosion is further noted. Note arrow depicts remaining inferior border of the mandible on CT and intra-operative image. On removal of the ramal prosthesis, extensive bony destruction is seen. It is caused by the polytetrafluoroethylene (PTFE, Proplast®), which is in direct contact with the lateral cortical bone.

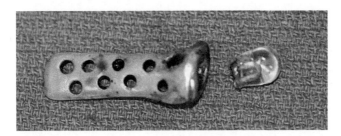

Figure 11.12 Fractured condylar head in type-I Christensen prosthesis. The type-I Christensen condylar prosthesis was made of chrome-cobalt-molybdenum alloy (Vitallium®) with a methyl-methacrylate head. It was associated with a high incidence of fracture and wear.

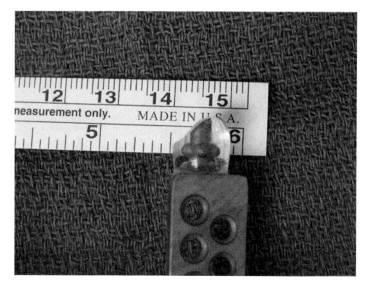

Figure 11.13 Flattened condylar head in type-II Christensen prosthesis. There were some minor design modifications seen from first to second generations of the Christensen prosthesis. However, the type-II Christensen condylar prosthesis, like the type I, was made of chrome-cobalt-molybdenum alloy (Vitallium®) body with a methyl-methacrylate head that was prone to wear with particulate debris and foreign body reaction.

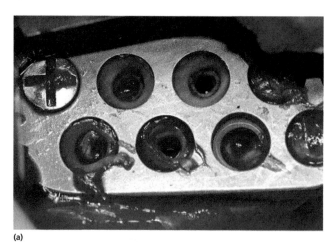

(a)

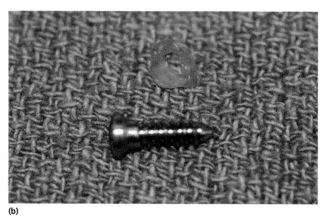

(b)

Figure 11.14 (a and b) Type-II Christensen prosthesis, granulation tissue surrounding screws used to fixate type-II Christensen prosthesis. There was gross mobility and lack of osseointegration with the ramus screws.

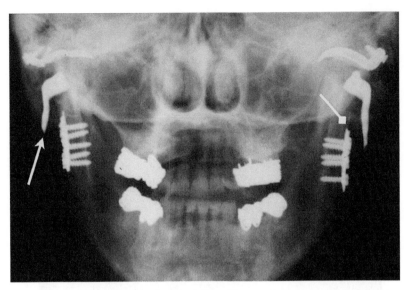

Figure 11.15 Posterior–anterior skull film showing bilateral fractured type-I Christensen prostheses (arrows). The increased thickness of the ramal strut with the offset design of the screw holes in the type-II Christensen prosthesis, which usually eliminated the problem of fracture, associated with the type-I Christensen prosthesis fractured at a point just above the most superior screws.

System were approved after premarket clinical trials.

Ankylosis

Ankylosis is clinically demonstrated as an inability to achieve adequate mouth opening, with subsequent difficulties in oral hygiene, mastication, and speech. The ankylotic bony mass often extends beyond the boundaries of the joint capsule. This presents three problems: (i) alteration of local anatomy and proximity to adjacent vasculature increases the risk of bleeding, (ii) increased bony mass renders the separation of the mandible from skull base more difficult and increases the risk of middle cranial fossa exposure or perforation, and (iii) limited movement of the mandible may cause fibrosis of musculature or elongation of the mandibular coronoid process, resulting in a secondary cause of trismus or persistent trismus if unaddressed. Intubation can be problematic with minimal mouth opening and necessitates fiberoptic intubation. Close communication and planning with the anesthesia team is essential for the safe induction of these patients. Additional anesthetic measures include awake intubation or tracheostomy when indicated.

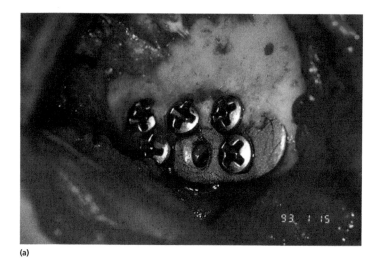

(a)

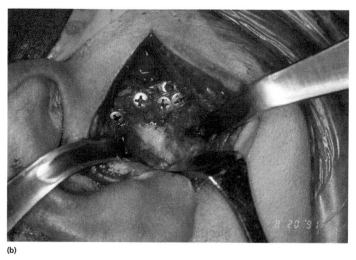

(b)

Figure 11.16 (a) Type-I Christensen prosthesis being submerged by heterotopic bone formation. This fixation of the prosthesis by bone served to create a stress point on the condylar prosthesis at the point where the bone formation ceased just above the most superior ramal screw. Fractures usually occurred at this point secondary to metal fatigue. (b) Heterotopic bone formation over a cast chrome-cobalt-molybdenum alloy Christensen fossa prosthesis that was placed against a natural condyle (hemiarthroplasty).

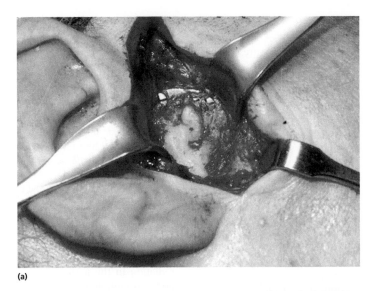

(a)

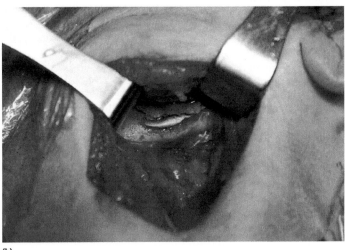

(b)

Figure 11.17 (a) Heterotopic bone formation encasing fossa component and (b) example of heterotopic bone evolving a mandibular prosthesis.

Summary

Surgical intervention is appropriate for a small percentage of patients with TMJ disorders. The decision to proceed should be based on a specific diagnosis of intracapsular pathology not responsive or amenable to nonsurgical treatment modalities. When TMJ surgery is considered, the potential complications and their management should be discussed with the patient.

Further reading

Carroll MJ. *et al.* (1987) Facial fractures in children. *Br Dent J,* 163:23.

Durr ED. *et al.* (1993) Radiation treatment of heterotopic bone formation in the temporomandibular articulation. Int J Radiat Oncol Biol Phys, 27:863–869.

Ellis E. *et al.* (1985) Ten years of mandibular fractures: an analysis of 2137 cases. *J Oral Surg,* 59:120.

Haug R. *et al.* (1990) An epidemiologic survey of facial fractures and concomitant injuries. *J Oral Maxillofac Surg,* 48:926.

Keith DA. (2003) Complications of temporomandibular joint surgery. *Oral Maxillofac Surg Clin North Am,* 15:187.

Kent JN. *et al.* (1986) Experience with a polymer glenoid fossa prosthesis for partial or total TMJ reconstruction. *J Oral Maxillofac Surg,* 44:520.

Kienapfel H. *et al.* (1999) Prevention of heterotopic bone formation after total hip arthroplasty. *Arch Orthop Trauma Surg,* 119:292–302.

Marker P. *et al.* (2000) Fractures of the mandibular condyle. Part I: patterns of distribution of types and causes of fractures in 348 patients. *Br J Oral Maxillofac Surg,* 38:417.

Mercuri LG. (2006) Microbial biofilms: a potential source of alloplastic device failure. *J Oral Maxillofac Surg,* 64:1303.

Mercuri LG, Anspach WE. (2003) Principles for the revision of total alloplastic TMJ prostheses. *Int J Oral Maxillofac Surg, 32*:353.

Neut D. *et al.* (2003) Detection of biomaterial-associated infections in orthopaedic joint implants. *Clin Orthop Relat Res,* 413:261.

Quinn PD. (2003) Alloplastic reconstruction of the temporomandibular joint. *Selected Readings Oral Maxillofac Surg,* 7:1–20.

Quinn PD. *et al.* (2006) Management of surgical failures. *Oral Maxillofac Surg Clin North Am,* 18:411.

Rees AM, Weinberg S. (1983) Fractures of the mandibular condyle: review of the literature and presentation of 5 cases with late complications. Surgical and nonsurgical correlations. *Oral Surg,* 73:37.

Reid R, Cooke H. (1999) Postoperative ionizing radiation in the management of heterotopic bone formation in the temporomandibular joint. *J Oral Maxillofac Surg,*57: 900–905.

Shaikh Z, Worrall S. (2002) Epidemiology of facial trauma in a sample of patients aged 1–18. *Injury,* 33:669.

Spagnoli D, Kent J. (1994) Alloplasts. *OMFS Knowledge Update,* 1.

Wolford LM, Karras SC. (1997) Autologous fat transplantation around temporomandibular joint total joint prostheses: preliminary treatment outcomes. *J Oral Maxillofac Surg,* 55:245–251.

Index

Note: Page numbers in *italics* refer to Figures; those in **bold** to Tables

alloplastic reconstruction
  custom prosthesis
    conjunction with orthognathic surgery, 181
    craniofacial deformity, 181
    orthognathic and TMJ prosthetic
      reconstruction, 187–200
    surgical planning *see* surgical planning
    wax-up of custom prosthesis, *184*, 187
  stock prosthesis
    advantages and disadvantages, 157
    alloplastic materials, 147
    autogenous joint replacement, 145
    bilateral ankylosis, *169, 170*
    Biomet stock prosthesis, 150–152, *160, 161*
    Christensen stock prosthesis, 148–50,
      154, 158
    class I occlusion, restoration, *170*
    complications, 166
    condylar prostheses, *147*, 147
    and custom alloplastic devices,
      comparison, **162**
    diamond rasp, *165, 166*
    3D reconstruction, *173*
    endotec prosthesis, *159*
    FDA-approved implants, 145, 169
    fossa and ramus prostheses, placement, *178*
    hemiarthroplasty, 155, *168*
    history, 146,` **146**
    ideal screw placement, 165
    indications, 145
    Kent-Vitek fossa, *150, 152*
    large condylar mass, *173*
    Lefort osteotomy, *177*
    osteochondroma, 172, *173, 174*
    osteotomy, *178*
    "plastic on metal" design, *159*
    potential interference evaluation, *177*
    preoperative planning, 157, 159
    "pseudo-translation," demonstration, *161*
    psoriatic arthritis, *176*
    Rasp overlying fossa, *160*
    reconstruction plate, *147, 148*
    "swan-neck" cervical deformity, *156, 162*
    two-step osteotomy, *163*, 163–4
ankylosis, *3*
  bilateral, *16, 169, 170, 185*
  bone scan, *27*
  bony, *98, 126*
  costochondral graft, 136–7
  eminoplasty, 94
  heterotopic bone formation, *243*
  imaging, *16, 27*
  intubation, 241
  oral hygiene, mastication and speech, 241
  problems, 241
  trismus and TMJ, *199–200*
  type-I Christensen prosthesis, *242*
arthritis
  psoriatic, *176*
  rheumatoid *see* rheumatoid arthritis
  septic *see* septic arthritis
  unilateral, *177*
arthrography
  ankylosis, pediatric patient, *13*
  bilateral degenerative joint disease, *12*
  "bird beaking" TMJ and condylar sclerosis, *12*
  bone windows, CT, *14*
  complications, 11

Atlas of Temporomandibular Joint Surgery, Second Edition. Edited by Peter D. Quinn and Eric J. Granquist.
© 2015 John Wiley & Sons, Inc. Published 2015 by John Wiley & Sons, Inc.
Companion Website: www.wiley.com/go/quinn/atlasTMJsurgery

arthrography (*cont'd*)
  condyle, osteoarthritis, *14*
  facial asymmetry, *14*
  "hoof" deformity, condylar head, *13*
  osteoarthritis, *13*
  videotaped arthrofluoroscopic study, 11
auricular cartilage
  disk replacement, 78
  graft harvesting, *79*
  post-meniscectomy, temporalis fascia graft, *81*
  temporalis muscle, myofascial or facial
    flap, *79, 80*
autogenous reconstruction
  advantages and disadvantages, 131
  costochondral graft, 131–8
  distraction osteogenesis, 139, 142–3
  vascularized (fibula) graft, 138–9

Biomet Microfixation TMJ Replacement
    System®, 237
Biomet stock prosthesis
  chrome–cobalt condylar prosthesis, 151
  condylar component, *162*
  fossa prosthesis, *160, 161*
  intermaxillary fixation, 151
  metal-on-x plastic design, 150
  microfixation, *195*
  placement, *161*
  total joint system, *160*
bone remodeling in children, 115, 129, *129*
bone scans
  ankylosis, *27*
  anterior joint space effusion, *27*
  radionucleotide imaging, *26, 27, 28*
  technetium-labeled phosphate complexes, *26*

chondrosarcomas
  malignant tumors, 228–9
  mesenchymal, 228
  synovial chondromatosis, *228*
Christensen stock prosthesis
  all-metallic version, *154, 158, 159*
  cobalt–chromium alloy fossa implant, 148–50
  natural condyle, *149*
  type-I Christensen prosthesis
    condylar, *149, 154, 157*
    fractured condylar head, *239*
    heterotopic bone formation, *242*
    posterior–anterior skull, *241*
  type-II-Christensen prosthesis
    condylar, *149, 154, 155, 156*
    flattened condylar head, *240*

Christensen TMJ Prosthesis System®, 237
complications
  ankylosis *see* ankylosis
  condylar fractures, 235–7
  hemorrhage, 233–4
  HTBF, 234
  infection, 234–5
  materials failure *see* materials failure
  nerve injury *see* nerve injury
computed tomography (CT)
  3D reconstruction and computer planning
    ankylosis, *16*
    bilateral condylar resorption, *18*
    bilateral sagittal fractures, condylar heads, *15*
    comminuted fracture, ramus and
      subcondylar region, *17*
    condylar displacement, *16*
    condylar head fracture, pediatric patient, *15*
    dislocated condyle, *16*
    maxilla and mandible repositioned, *18*
    septic arthritis, *17*
    three-dimensional CT images, *19*
  temporomandibular region, imaging,
    111–12, *114*
condylar diskopexey *see* diskopexey
condylar fractures, 3
  bilateral, 109
  in children
    degree of fracture displacement, 129
    detection, 123
    follow-up program, 130
    incidence, 123
    physical and radiographic examination, 126
  head fracture, *15, 110, 111*
condylar hyperplasia, 27, *28, 213, 214*, 224–5
condylectomy
  bone-holding forceps, *98*
  condyle sectioning, 100
  Dunn-Dautrey retractors, 99–100, *96*
  extensive posttraumatic bony ankylosis, *98*
  fissure bur, *97*
  modified posterior mandibular incision, 99
  osteotomies sequence, *99*
  prosthesis/costochondral graft, 99
  retromandibular incision, 100
  spring-loaded bell exerciser, *99*
  standard endaural approach, 99, *96*
  T-bar osteotome, 100, *97*
condyloplasty, 57, 63, 85, *86*
condylotomy
  advantages, 103
  chronic TMJ pain, 103

condyle ramus complex, *101*
   disadvantages, 103
   intraoral coronoidectomy, *102*
   modified, 82
   proximal segment, 103
   ward, *100–102*
coronoidectomy, *102, 159, 167*
costochondral graft
   ankylosis, 136
   complications, 138
   "double stacked," *136*
   endaural incision, *134,* 135
   function and adaptation, *137*
   in glenoid fossa, *137*
   harvested costochondral graft, *136*
   hemifacial microsomia, *135,* 135
   heterotopic bone formation, 131–2
   hyaline cartilage, *133,* 134–5
   intermaxillary fixation, 135, 136
   multiple fragments, *134*
   in pediatric patients, 131
   with perichondrium intact, *133*
   placement, *132*
   resection of osteochondroma, *138*
   retromandibular incision, *135*
   ribs, harvesting, *132, 132–3, 133, 136*
custom cutting guides, *193*

decision making, 1–4
Delrin-Timesh condylar prosthesis, *147, 151*
dermal graft, 78
desmoplastic fibroma, 219
discectomy *see* meniscectomy
diskopexey
   description, 71
   displaced disk deformation, *74*
   meniscal repositioning, *72*
   Mitek anchoring system, 71, *73*
   nonresorbable suture, *72*
   stage III and stage IV internal
      derangements, 71
disk plication
   description, 69
   disk repositioning, posterior attachment, *70*
   eminoplasty, chronic open lock
      treatment, *70*
   modified right-angle vascular clamps, 69
   repositioned meniscus, *69*
distraction osteogenesis
   advances in multidirectional distractors and
      CT planning, 142
   advantages, 139

challenges and complications, 139
   device placement, *143*
Dunn-Dautrey retractors, *96, 99–100,* 164

eminoplasty
   articular eminence, medial extent, *91*
   bone file, 86
   bony perforations and status post, *92*
   condylar head and glenoid fossa cryosection, *87*
   CT and MRI, 85, *94*
   Dautrey procedure, articular eminence, *95*
   dislocation, *87, 88*
   glenoid fossa with eminence reduced, *89*
   high condylar shave, *86*
   hypermobility treatment, 85
   inadvertent ankylosis, 94
   lateral cortical, *91*
   mandible, unobstructed condylar motion, *93*
   middle cranial fossa, proximity, *90*
   osteotomy, *89, 90*
   persistent dislocation, emergency room
      intervention, *93*
   rasp, *92*
   subluxation, 85
endaural incision
   description, 39–40
   placement, *38, 39*
   vs. preauricular approach, *44*
   retraction, skin flap, *43*
   well-healed, *48, 52*
exophytic osteoma, *217*
extra-abdominal desmoid, 219
extraoral technique, *121*
extraoral vertical ramus osteotomy, *214*

facial nerve
   frontal and zygomatic branches, *43, 232*
   galvanic stimulation, 33
   main trunk identification, *33*
   normal condyle and fossa, mandible closed, *32*
   permanent nerve damage, 33
   postsurgical palsy, 33
   from stylomastoid foramen, *32*
   temporal branch, 31, 38, *42, 47, 223,* 231
fibromatosis, aggressive
   description, 219
   diagnosis, 220
fixation techniques, 121
   intermaxillary fixation, Risdon wire, *128*
   methods, 117–23
   rigid fixation, 115–16, *118*
   skeletal fixation, nasal spine wire, *127*

foreign body reactions
  clinical and radiographic examinations, 225
  displaced condyle, *226*
  exophytic preauricular mass, *228*
  irregular spicule of bone, *227*
  osteogenic sarcoma, *227*
  palpable exophytic mass, *226*
  proplast (polytetraflouroethylene), 225
  Teflon-proplast implant, 225

giant cell tumor
  axial and coronal condyle, *218*
  postresection, *219*
  surgical specimen, *218*
glenoid fossa
  costochondral graft, *137*
  cryosection, *87*
  fracture, *124*
  middle cranial fossa fenestration, *187*
Goldenhar syndrome, *205*
"green stick" fractures, 108, 126

hemarthrosis, *108*
hemiarthroplasty or partial joint
      reconstruction, *149*, 155, *168, 242*
heterotopic bone formation (HTBF), 82, 155,
      166, *183*, 234, 242, 243
"hoof" deformity, *13, 206*
hypermobility, *4, 85*

imaging
  arthrography, 11, *12–14*
  bone scans, 26–8
  computer tomography (CT), 14–19
  magnetic resonance imaging (MRI), 19–26
  orthopantogram, 5–6
  plain film radiography, 5, 7, *113*
  tomograms, 5–11
internal derangements, surgery, 2
  anteriorly displaced disk without reduction, *65*
  anterior-medially displaced disk and tissue
      forceps, *68*
  articular eminence, 62
  #15 blade, 57–9
  Cadaver specimen, condyle and dissected
      disk, *63*
  capsule extent, *58*
  condyle in open position, *68*
  condyloplasty, 63, 66
  direct trauma prevention, 63
  diskopexey *see* diskopexey

disk plication *see* disk plication
disk position evaluation, 59
endaural approach, *66*
incision into inferior joint space, *60*
joint capsule incision and superior joint
      space, 59
lateral pterygoid with fat plane separation, *62*
meniscal salvage procedures, 57
meniscectomy *see* meniscectomy
meniscoplasty, *68, 70*
modified condylotomy, 82
MRI, 20
open joint procedures, 57
physiologic position, meniscus, *67*
postoperative care, 82, *82, 83*
reciprocal clicking, *64*
repair/meniscectomy, disk isolation, *60*
superior joint space, *62*
TMJ capsule, 59
T1 MRI closed and open positions, *64, 65*
Wilkes classification, **58**
Wilkes retractor, *61, 66*
intracapsular fracture, *111*

jaw exercise physical therapy, *129*

Kent-Vitek Prosthesis (VK-I)
  bilaminate glenoid fossa implant, 237
  mandibular component, *152*
  ramus prosthesis, *153*
  removal, *152*
  synthes reconstruction plate, *150*
  total joint prosthesis, *152*
K-wire, *118, 121*

lag-screw-washer technique, *118,* 119, *123*
Lefort osteotomy, *175, 176*
Lefort 1 osteotomy, *198*

magnetic resonance imaging (MRI)
  anteriorly displaced disk, *21, 23, 24, 25*
  closed mouth T1 MRI, left TMJ, *22*
  condyle disk position, *20, 21*
  degenerative condylar changes and meniscus
      thinning, *25*
  degenerative joint disease, *26*
  disk and capsule attachments, *26*
  disk displacement, 20
  ferromagnetic clips, 19
  lateral disk herniation, *26*
  retrodiscal tissue thickening, *23*

T1 and T2 weighted images, 19
temporomandibular region, 111–12, *114*
mandibular condyle fractures
    classification
        anatomic location and condylar fragment,
            112, 115
        type I fracture (nondisplaced), 115
        type II fracture (fracture deviation), 115
        type III fracture (fracture displacement), 115
        type IV fracture (fracture dislocation), 115
    signs and symptoms, 109–10
    treatment
        alternative shaped plates, *119*
        bone remodeling in children, 115
        bony ankylosis, *126*
        in children, 123–30, *127*
        closed treatment, 116
        condylar fractures, *125*
        displaced condylar head, *124, 128*
        extraoral technique, *121*
        fixation techniques, 121
        glenoid fossa, fracture, *124*
        intermaxillary fixation, Risdon wire, *128*
        internal fixation, 115
        jaw exercise physical therapy, *129*
        lag screw technique, *123*
        "lamda" plate, 120
        methods of fixation, 117–23
        open reduction, **116,** 116–17
        rigid fixation, 115–16, *118*
        skeletal fixation, nasal spine wire, *127*
        "square" plate configuration, *118, 119*
        stabilizing condylar fractures, *118*
        subcondylar fracture, *120, 122*
materials failure
    Dacron-reinforced silicone sheet, *238*
    failed fibula reconstruction, *238*
    foreign-body giant cell reaction, *238*
    Kent-Vitek Prosthesis (VK-I), *237, 239*
    polytetrafluoroethylene, 237
    posterior-anterior skull film, *241*
    TMJ replacement systems, 237, 241
    type-I Christensen prosthesis, *239*
    type-II Christensen prosthesis, *240*
    types, 237
    UHMWPE, 237
maxillofacial radiographic technique, 110
meniscectomy
    crepitus, 75, 77
    curved TMJ scissors, 74
    description, 74

disk thinning and perforation, 74, *75*
medical-grade silicone sheeting, 77
postauricular approach, *77*
with replacement
    auricular cartilage *see* auricular cartilage
    autogenous, allogeneic and alloplastic
        materials, 78
    dermal graft, 78
    temporalis muscle and fascial grafts, 81
retained foreign bodies, 78
temporary silastic implant, *76, 77*
meniscoplasty
    anterior-medially displaced meniscus, *68*
    disk repositioning, *70*
    open joint procedures, 57
Mitek anchoring system, 71, *73*
Mitek bone-cleat introducer, 71
MRI *see* magnetic resonance imaging (MRI)

neoplasms, **204,** 228–9
nerve injury
    condylectomy/screw placement, 232
    cranial nerves V and VII, 231
    galvanic stimulation, 232
    hematoma with endaural approach, *232*
    necrosis of skin flap, *232*
    neuropraxia, 231
    ophthalmic drops, 231–2
    orbicularis oculi, 231
    periprosthetic soft tissue, *233*
    postsurgical keloid, *233*
    postsurgical palsy, 231
    risk of nerve damage, 231
    TMJ surgery, 231
    trigeminal nerve branches, 232
    zygomatic branches, 231, *232*

oculo-auricular-vertebral syndrome, *205*
orthognathic and TMJ prosthetic
        reconstruction
    abdominal fat graft, *190*
    absolute trismus and TMJ ankylosis, *199–200*
    Biomet microfixation, *195*
    computer aid modeling, *191*
    computer-generated fossa design, *191*
    custom cutting guides, *193*
    3D stereo laser model, patient's anatomy, *189*
    final custom prosthesis design, *191*
    infected custom metal-on-metal alloplastic
        total joint, *194*
    maxillary osteotomy, *192*

oculo-auricular-vertebral syndrome (*cont'd*)
  postoperative panorex and prosthesis
      planned positioning, *196*
  prediction and radiographic tracing, *189*
  presurgery lateral cephalogram, *189*
  ramus reconstruction, *189*
  rhabdomyosarcoma, resection and radiation,
      197–9
  stages, surgical procedures, *188*
  trial fossa component, *191, 192*
orthopantogram radiography, 5–6
osseous surgery
  condylectomy *see* condylectomy
  condyloplasty, 85
  condylotomy, 103
  eminoplasty *see* eminoplasty
osteochondroma
  facial asymmetry, *215, 216*
  laterognathia, *215*
  reconstruction with stock alloplastic total
      joint, *216*
  temporomandibular joint and resection, *216*
osteotomy
  articular eminence, *89*
  condylar neck, *99, 182*
  Dunn-Dautrey retractors, *96*
  extraoral vertical ramus, *214*
  internal maxillary artery, *96, 97, 99, 164*
  intra-oral vertical ramus, 103, 119
  intraoral vertical subsigmoid, *82, 82, 103,*
      213, 225
  Lefort 1, *198*
  mandibular repositioning, 183
  two-step, 100, *163,* 163–4
  vertical subcondylar, *102*

pathology
  benign tumors *see* tumors
  foreign body reactions, 225–6
  malignant tumors *see* tumors
  rheumatoid arthritis *see* rheumatoid arthritis
  septic arthritis *see* septic arthritis
pigmented villonodular synovitis, *223*
plain film radiography, 5, 7, *113*
polytetrafluoroethylene (PTFE), 77, 78,
      237, *239*
Proplast®, 237, *239*

retromandibular surgical approach
  anatomic structures, *49*
  blunt dissection, 48

curved hemostat, *46*
dissection, facial and periosteum, *45*
facial nerve monitoring, *43*
fascial layers and facial nerve,
      temporoparietal fascial, *47*
mandible exposure, *51*
marginal mandibular branch, 48
marking, modified, *49*
masseter exposed, *51*
nerve stimulator, 48
parotidectomy and extended preauricular
      incision combination, *42*
Risdon submandibular approach, 45
submandibular gland and posterior belly, *50*
superficial temporal artery and vein, *42*
temporomandibular joint capsule exposure, *45*
well-healed, *52*
rheumatoid arthritis
  bilateral total joint reconstruction and
      anterior open bite closure, *211*
  psoriatic, *211*
  surgical algorithms, 203
  temporary cessation, coordination, 204
rhytidectomy, 31, 39, 41, 117

sarcoma
  osteogenic, *226, 227, 229, 227*
  synovial, 228
septic arthritis, *4*
  acute degeneration, condyle, *210*
  anterior open bite and progressive joint
      pain, *210*
  description, 204
  displacement of condyle, *17, 19*
  hemifacial microsomia with auricular
      defect, *205*
  "Hoof" deformity, *206*
  hypoplastic left condyle from early condylar
      trauma, *205*
  imaging, 204
  initial aspiration, joint for cytology and
      culture, *209*
  interpositional implant, *207*
  normal class-1 occlusion, *210*
  normal pain-free function, *210*
  panorex demonstration, *209*
  preauricular swelling, *208*
  rim enhancement, *208*
subcondylar fractures, *107*
  bilateral, *113, 120*
  displaced, *107, 110, 120*

surgical approaches
  decision making, 1–4
  endaural, 39–40
  for internal derangements *see* internal
      derangements, surgery
  intraoral, *52, 53*
  postauricular, *40, 40–41, 41*
  preauricular, *38, 38–9, 44*
  prep and positioning, 53, *54, 55*
  retromandibular *see* retromandibular surgical
      approach
  rhytidectomy, 41
surgical planning
  advantages, 187
  anatomic models, 182–3
  bilateral complete bony TMJ ankylosis, *185*
  bilateral TMJ replacement, *186*
  computer modeling, 183, 187
  disadvantages, 183, 187
  fossa and condylar components, *182*
  initial prosthesis design, *184*
  intraoperative imaging, *182*
  joint replacement prior to implantation, *182*
  malocclusion, *184*
  preoperative 3D reconstruction, 183, *181*
  prepubertal bilateral mandibular condyle
      fractures, *185*
  pure titanium mesh backing, *186*
  stage 1 bilateral gap arthroplasties, *185*
  temporal-zygomatic bone loss, *186*
  two-piece stereolithic model, 183, *181, 184*
  wax-up of prosthesis, *184*
"swan-neck" cervical deformity, *156, 162*
synovial chondromatosis
  axial MRI, *221*
  cartilaginous metaplasia, 213
  chondrosarcomas, *228*
  MRI images, *220*
  skull invasion, *222*

T-bar osteotomes, *97, 100*
Teflon®-coated fluoroethyl polyethylene
    (FEP), 237
Teflon/proplast implants
  with fragmentation and wear evident, *207*
  giant cell reaction, *208*
  interpositional implant, *207*
  packaging and demonstration, *206*
  perforated, *208*
temporomandibular joint (TMJ) surgery
  complications *see* complications

Kent-Vitek Prosthesis (VK-I), 237
patients, 243
postsurgical infections, 234
TheraBite jaw exerciser, *83*
third-body wear phenomenon, 146
TMJ Concepts® Prosthesis, 237
Trauma
  bilateral condylar fractures, 109
  bilateral subcondylar fractures, *113, 120*
  3D reconstruction, *113*
  "green stick" fractures, 108, 126
  hemarthrosis, *108*
  incidence, 106
  intracapsular fracture, *111*
  ipsilateral condylar fracture, 107
  mandibular condyle fractures
      classification, 112–15
      signs and symptoms, 109–10
      treatment, 115–16
  mechanism of injury, 106–8
  subcondylar fracture, *107*
  symphyseal or parasymphyseal fracture, 107
  temporomandibular region, imaging
      computed tomography (CT), 111–12, *114*
      magnetic resonance imaging (MRI),
          111–12, *114*
      maxillofacial radiographic technique, 110
trigeminal nerve
  auriculotemporal nerve, 33, *34*
  foramen ovale position, *34*
  inferior alveolar branch, 35
  superficial temporal artery and vein, *35*
tumors
  benign
      acute-onset condylar hyperplasia, *213*
      aggressive fibromatosis, 219–20
      cephalometric and panorex postoperative, *214*
      chin midline and with good joint function, *217*
      condylar hyperplasia and good joint
          function, *214*
      CT and MRI scans, 219
      exophytic osteoma, *217*
      extraoral vertical ramus osteotomy, *214*
      facial asymmetry and laterognathia, *215*
      giant cell granulomas, 211
      giant cell tumor *see* giant cell tumor
      gross distension, *220*
      hemimandibular hypertrophy, *212*
      histologic events, 224
      intraoral vertical subsigmoid osteotomy
          genioplasty, *213*

maxillary midline, *215*
meniscectomy, 219
normal condyle with degenerative
   condyle, *212*
osteochondroma *see* osteochondroma
osteoma excision, *218*
preoperative and postoperative occlusion, *217*
progressive facial asymmetry and
   malocclusion, *215*
synovial chondromatosis, 213
unilateral open bite, *212*
malignant
   chondrosarcomas, 228
   description, 228
   malignancy affecting skeletal bones, 229
   medial aspect, condyle, *229*
   paresthesia, 229

ultra-high-molecular-weight polyethylene
   (UHMWPE), 146, 237

vascular anatomy
   condylectomy, 35
   external carotid artery, 35
   external maxillary artery isolation, *37*
   maxillary artery and branches, *36*
   osteotomies, *36*
vascularized (fibula) graft
   complications, *142*
   failed hardware and mandibular
      defect, *140*
   fibula free flap, 138, *139*
   free fibular graft, *140*
   functional status and skeletal
      symmetry, *141*
   postoperative physical therapy, 139
   virtual surgical planning, *141*
vertical dimension of occlusion (VDO), *167*
Vitallium®, *239, 240*

Wilkes classification, **58**, *61, 66*

Printed and bound by CPI Group (UK) Ltd, Croydon, CR0 4YY

16/04/2025

14658459-0001